Therapeutic Angiography

Edited by
C. A. Athanasoulis
H. L. Abrams   E. Zeitler

Contributors
K. Amplatz · K.H. Barth · J.J. Bookstein · D.C. Brewster · V.P. Chuang
A.M. Cohen · R.F. Colapinto · A.B. Cosimi · N.P. Couch · V. DeCaprio
J.L. Doppman · C.T. Dotter · E.J. Ferris · A.J. Greenfield
E.P. Harries-Jones · I. Iossifides · I.S. Johnsrude · K.W. Johnston
S.L. Kaufmann · F.S. Keller · R.A. Malt · M.F. Mozes · D.C. Nabseth
R.A. Novelline · A.M. Palestrant · K. Pringle · J. Rösch · W. Rösch
A.H. Robbins · D.E. Schwarten · G.V. Segre · M. Simon · E.E. Slater
D.G. Spigos · J.D. Strandberg · W.S. Tan · W.M. Thompson · S. Wallace
A.C. Waltman · C. Wang · R.I. White, Jr. · W.C. Widrich · E. Zeitler

With 75 Figures

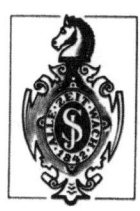

Springer-Verlag
Berlin Heidelberg New York 1981

CHRISTOS A. ATHANASOULIS, M.D.
Department of Radiology, Harvard Medical School, Massachusetts General Hospital, Fruit Street, Boston, MA 02115, USA

HERBERT L. ABRAMS, M.D.
Department of Radiology, Harvard Medical School, 25 Shattuck Street, Boston, MA 02115, USA

EBERHARD ZEITLER, Prof. Dr.
Klinikum Nürnberg, Radiologisches Zentrum, Flurstraße 17, D-8500 Nürnberg

This monograph comprises number 4 (volume 3) of the Springer journal *Cardiovascular and Interventional Radiology*.

ISBN 978-3-540-10526-8   ISBN 978-3-642-95382-8 (eBook)
DOI 10.1007/978-3-642-95382-8

Offsetprinting and Binding: Universitätsdruckerei H. Stürtz AG, Würzburg
2127/3130-543210

Preface

Applications of angiography have expanded to include not only diagnostic procedures but also therapeutic interventions. The introduction of regional administration of vasoactive drugs through percutaneously placed angiographic catheters was soon followed by methods of transcatheter vessel occlusion using temporary or permanent embolic materials. At the same time methods of opening up narrowed or completely obstructed blood vessels with percutaneously introduced balloon catheters were being perfected. Thus, regional blood flow reduction or regional blood flow increase can now be accomplished with percutaneous angiographic methods in lieu of major surgical interventions. The advantages in terms of reduced morbidity, length of hospital stay and cost are evident.

Therapeutic angiography is a rapidly advancing and therefore changing field. This monograph aims at capturing some of the most recent advances and also at presenting some of the controversies. In order to accomplish this task the editors invited a selected group of cardiovascular radiologists, to contribute in their respective fields of therapeutic angiography. For a balanced view other experts – usually nonradiologists – were also asked to present their views, comments, and criticisms. Whenever opinions were far apart an opportunity was given for reply or rebuttal. Thus, up-to-date information with supporting or opposing expert views is presented on the topics of transluminal angioplasty, transcatheter vessel occlusion, regional drug infusions, and radiologic interventions in thromboembolic disease.

The editors wish to thank the authors for their excellent contributions and hope that the reader will find this monograph informative, practical, and useful in the clinical application of therapeutic angiography.

January 1981

CHRISTOS A. ATHANASOULIS, M.D.
Department of Radiology
Harvard Medical School
Massachusetts General Hospital
Boston, MA

Contents

Percutaneous Transluminal Angioplasty of the Renal Artery

Donald E. Schwarten

Department of Radiology, St. Vincent Hospital and Health Care Center, Indianapolis, Indiana, USA

Abstract. Percutaneous transluminal renal angioplasty (PTRA) has been employed in 70 renal arteries, utilizing the balloon angioplasty technique described by Grüntzig for peripheral vessels. The procedure has been employed both in patients with normal renal function and in selected patients with decreased renal function. The complication rate has been low (5.7%), and no patient has required operative intervention as a result of a complication sustained during PTRA. The early results of PTRA compare favorably to those achieved through operative revascularization. An assessment of the duration of PTRA's effects must however, await the results of long-term follow-up.

Key words: Renal arteries – Angioplasty – Catheters and catheterization – Interventional radiology.

Approximately 5% of hypertensive individuals in the United States have renovascular hypertension, and, therefore, a correctable cause for their disease. However, in this high-risk group of patients who frequently have generalized arteriosclerotic disease, surgical correction is associated with relatively high mortality [1], as well as significant morbidity and loss of productive work time. Medical management, though it is without these immediate drawbacks, is associated with a much lower long-term survival rate than is surgery [2]. Revascularization techniques, as developed by Dotter [3] and refined by Grüntzig [4–7], offer the possibility of renal artery stenosis correction via percutaneous transluminal renal angioplasty techniques (PTRA) (Fig. 1).

During the past 22 months we have applied the principles of PTRA to 70 renal arteries in patients

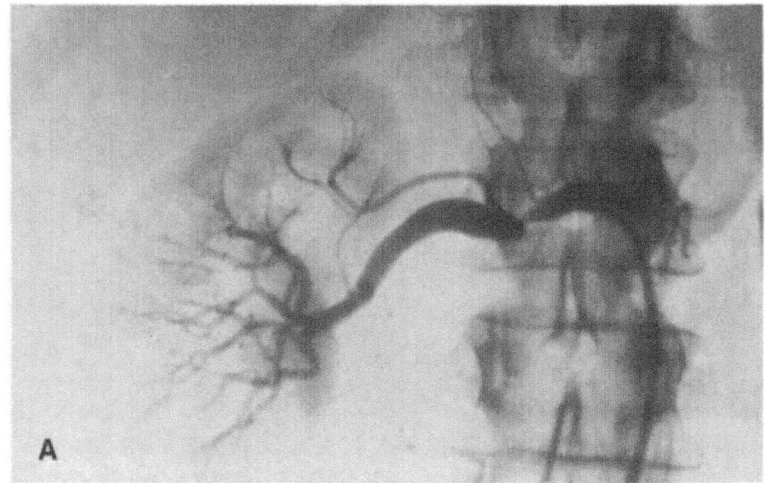
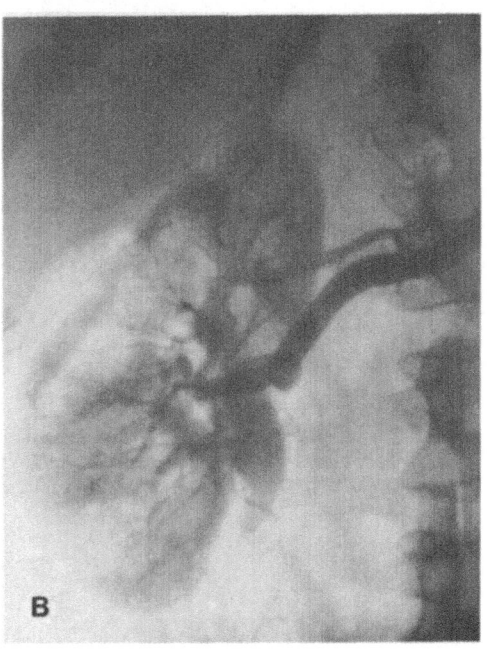

Fig. 1 A and B. Pre-PTRA (**A**) and post-PTRA (**B**) arteriograms.

Address reprint requests to: D.E. Schwarten, M.D., Department of Radiology, St. Vincent Hospital and Health Care Center, 2001 W. 86th Street, Indianapolis, IN 46260, USA

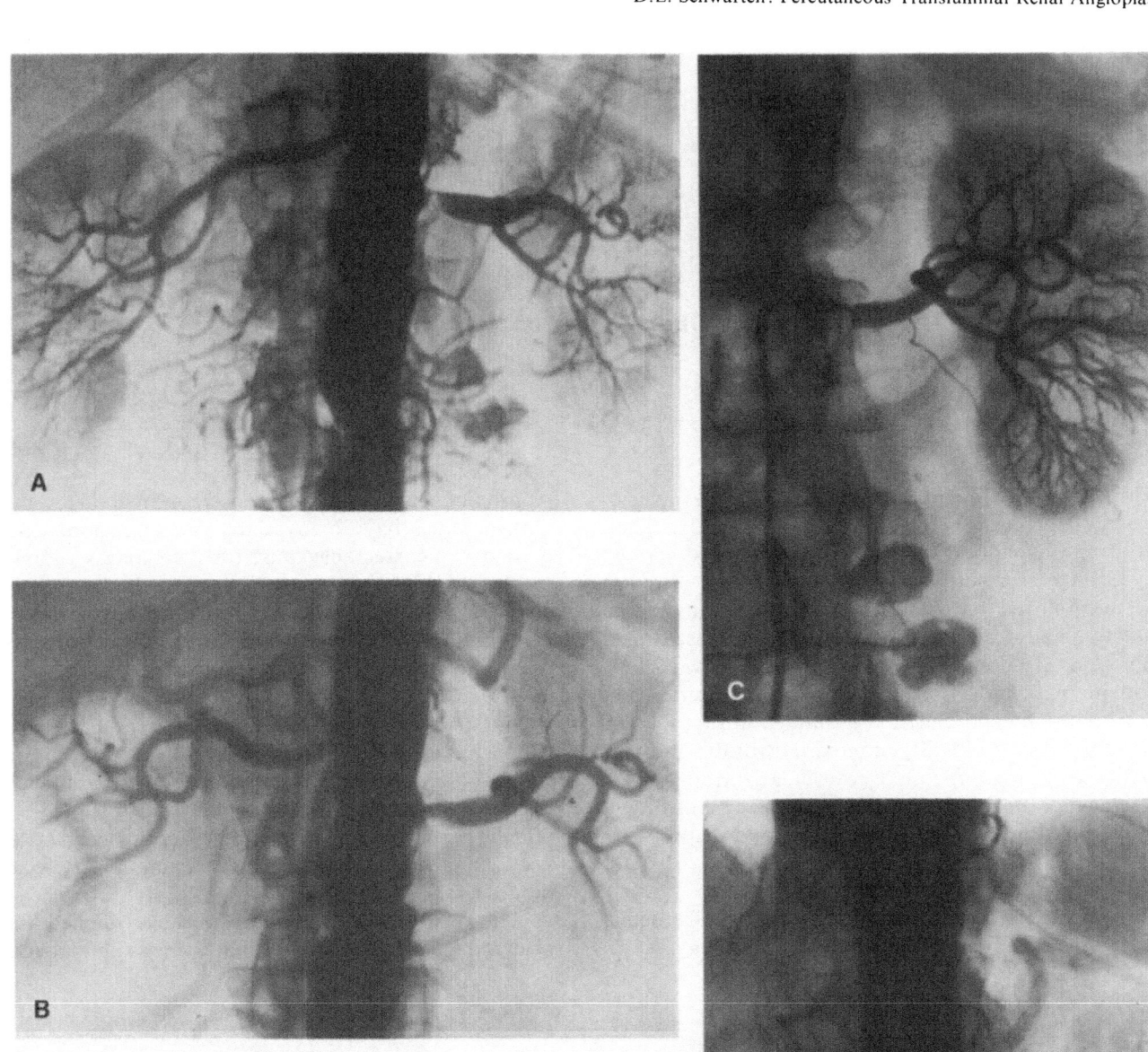

Fig. 2A–D. Arteriographic studies of a patient is whom repeat PTRA was performed for recurrent renal artery stenosis after an initial PTRA procedure. Initial PTRA: pre-PTRA (**A**) and post-PTRA (**B**) arteriograms. Repeat PTRA nine months after initial procedure: pre-PTRA (**C**) and post-PTRA (**D**) arteriograms.

with renovascular hypertension for correction of renal artery stenosis and/or preservation of renal function. Patients who have undergone PTRA, for the most part, would have been candidates for the classical operative renal revascularization.

Materials and Methods

Patients

Percutaneous transluminal angioplasty was performed in three groups with renal artery stenosis:

Group 1. Patients with refractory hypertension and a renin vein ratio of 1.5 to 1 or greater (38 patients).

Group 2. Patients with refractory hypertension who did not show lateralization of renin values (22 patients).

Group 3. Patients with a solitary kidney with azotemia and rapidly deteriorating renal function, with or without hypertension (two patients); and patients with hypertension with azotemia, decreasing renal function, and bilateral renal artery stenoses (10 patients).

The use of PTRA was not ruled out in cases in which lateralizing renin values were not found if there was severe renal artery stenosis and uncontrollable hypertension, since reports have indicated the possibility of improvement in blood pressure control despite the lack of lateralization of renin values [8, 9] and because prevention of renal artery occlusion seemed desirable.

The renal artery stenosis was due to atherosclerosis in all but five of the 70 patients treated. In the remaining five, medial disease was responsible for the stenosis.

Technique

The PTRA technique employed, which has been described by Katzen [10], is a modification of Grüntzig's method. After a preshaped catheter was selectively introduced into the renal artery, a small guidewire, inserted through the catheter, was advanced beyond the renal artery stenosis. The catheter was then exchanged over the guidewire for a Grüntzig catheter of appropriate balloon diameter, which was placed in the stenotic area. The balloon was then inflated. After completion of the dilatation, pressure measurements were obtained and angiography performed.

Anti-hypertensive medications were discontinued 48 hours before PTRA, if possible. If blood pressure control was a problem, short-acting agents such as nitroprusside, were used. Administration of medication to prevent platelet aggregation (650 mg of aspirin and 50 mg of persantine twice a day) was begun 24 hours before the revascularization. Systemic heparinization was employed during the procedure.

Patients were carefully monitored for the first 24 hours after PTRA because of the possibility of profound changes in blood pressure occurring over very brief periods of time.

Results

In 93% of the cases in which it was performed, PTRA met with early success; in one patient who sustained a minor intimal injury during selective catheterization, angioplasty was not attempted. PTRA was not successful in four cases, one in which the catheter could not be introduced into the stenotic area, and three in which the stenosis was not satisfactorily dilated.

Four of the initial successes have gone on to restenosis within one year after PTRA. Their angiographic appearance differed from that of the initial typical atherosclerotic lesion (Fig. 2), in that the restenoses appeared to conform to the total area in contact with the balloon during the dilatation. Two of the patients with restenosis have undergone uneventful repeat PTRA, which was more easily performed than was the initial procedure.

In the patients with chemically proven renin-dependent hypertension (Group 1) the average blood pressure readings dropped dramatically following successful PTRA, paralleling the changes in renal vein renin values. Before PTRA the average blood pressure in Group 1 was 190/110 mm Hg; 48 hours after PTRA, the average blood pressure was 135/70 mm Hg (Fig. 3). The patients with the greatest renin dependency exhibited the most profound decrease in blood pressure. Medication requirements also decreased in this group. Before PTRA, patients had had poor control of blood pressure despite an average intake of 3.1 antihypertensive medications per patient, while after the procedure their blood pressures had normalized on an average of 0.5 medications per patient. At six months 90% of the Group 1 patients were considered cured or improved, and in 10% the procedure was considered a failure.

The results in patients without lateralization of renin values (Group 2), while not as dramatic as in patients in Group 1, were gratifying. In this group the average blood pressure decreased from 200/100 mm Hg to 140/85 mm Hg after PTRA, and medication requirements also decreased (Fig. 4).

Patients with compromised renal function who underwent PTRA for preservation of renal function as well as for control of hypertension (Group 3) had the least gratifying results, both immediately and over the long-term (Fig. 5). The effects of PTRA on renal function in these patients, while similarly suboptimal, were considered successful in light of the underlying disease process in most of these patients. The majority of these patients have now passed the one year follow-up period, and renal function has stabilized rather than deteriorated. Two patients in Group 3 were in acute renal failure, and it is these two patients that skew the curve because of their dramatic response to PTRA both in terms of blood pressure response and renal function.

Complications occurred in 5.7% of procedures, but no patient in this series sustained a complication

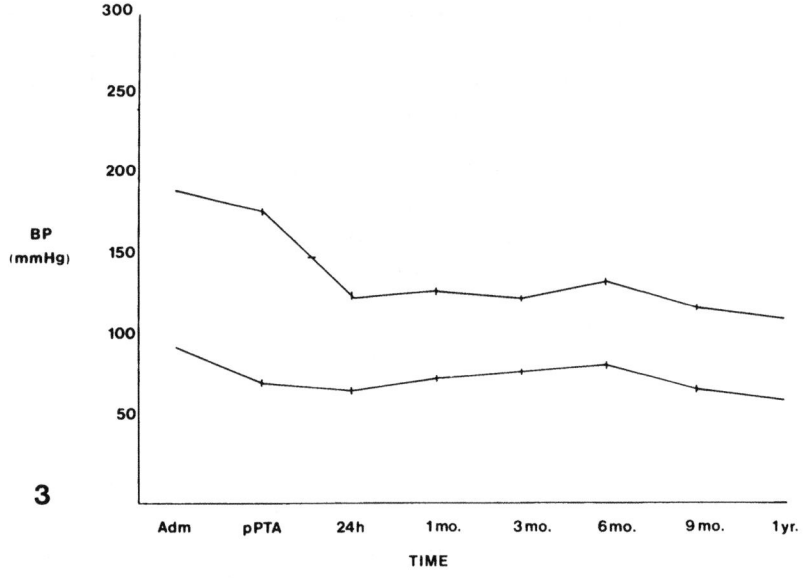

3

Fig. 3. Average blood pressure response to PTRA in patients with renin-dependent hypertension.

Fig. 4. Average blood pressure response in patients with renal artery stenosis, but no proof of renin lateralization.

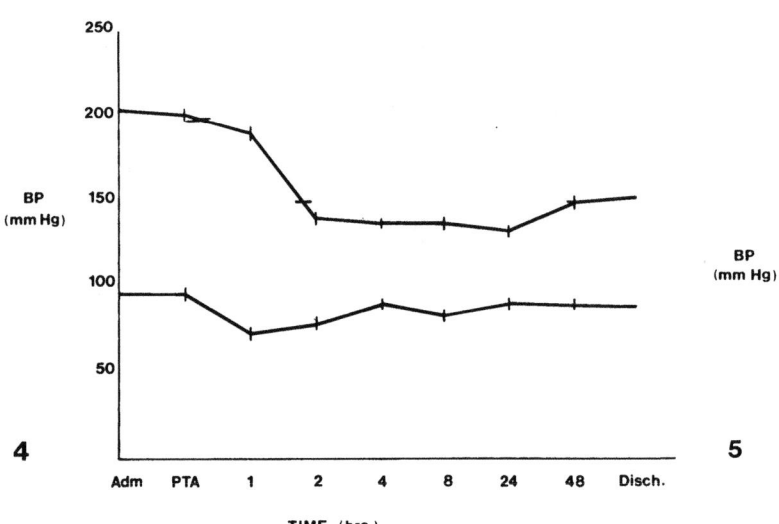

4

5

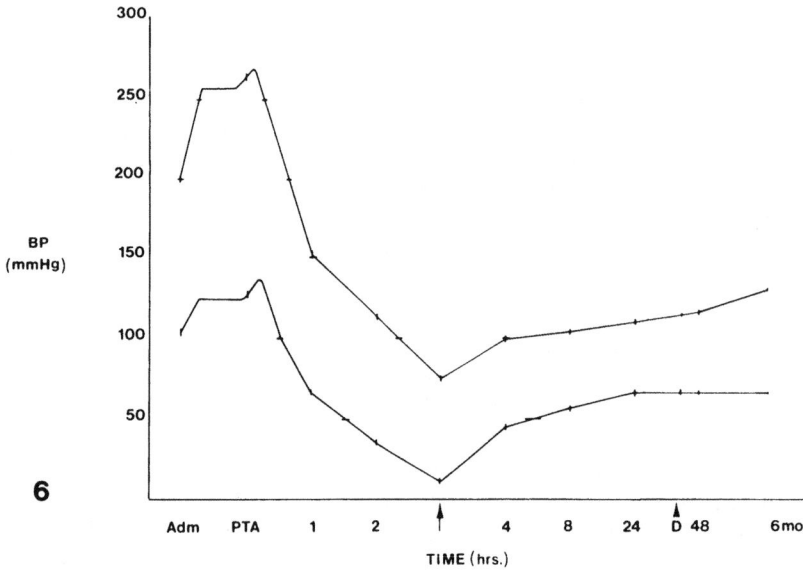

6

Fig. 5. Average blood pressure response in patients with renal failure. Peak at three months is due to recurrent stenosis in one patient.

Fig. 6. Blood pressure response manifested by patient whose arteriographic studies are shown in Figure 2. *Arrow* indicates onset of dopamine infusion. *D* indicates cessation of dopamine infusion.

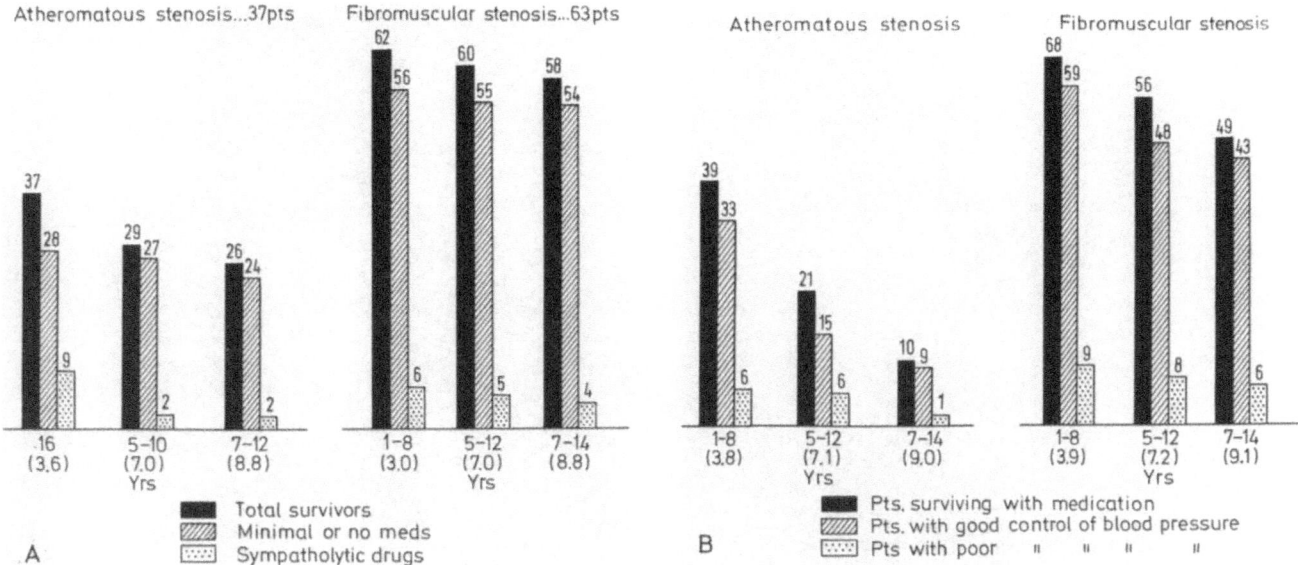

Atheromatous stenosis...37pts
Fibromuscular stenosis...63pts
37 28 9
29 27 2
26 24 2
62 56 6
60 55 5
58 54 4
16 (3.6)
5-10 (7.0)
7-12 (8.8)
Yrs
1-8 (3.0)
5-12 (7.0)
7-14 (8.8)
Yrs
Total survivors
Minimal or no meds
Sympatholytic drugs
A
Atheromatous stenosis
Fibromuscular stenosis
39 33 6
21 15 6
10 9 1
68 59 9
56 48 8
49 43 6
1-8 (3.8)
5-12 (7.1)
7-14 (9.0)
Yrs
1-8 (3.9)
5-12 (7.2)
7-14 (9.1)
Yrs
Pts. surviving with medication
Pts. with good control of blood pressure
Pts with poor " " " "
B

Fig. 7 A and B. Comparative survivals in renovascular hypertension with surgical (**A**) vs. medical (**B**) management. (Data obtained from [2].)

A
B

C

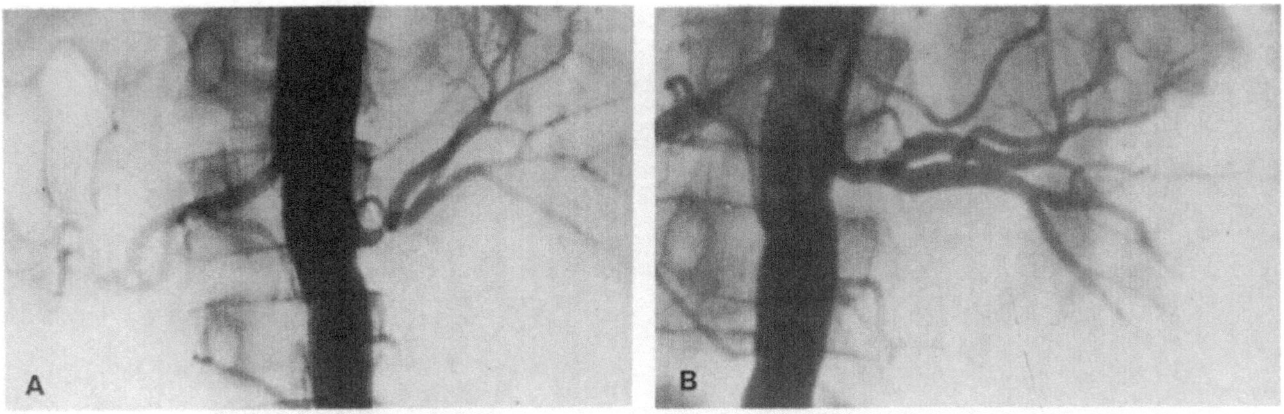

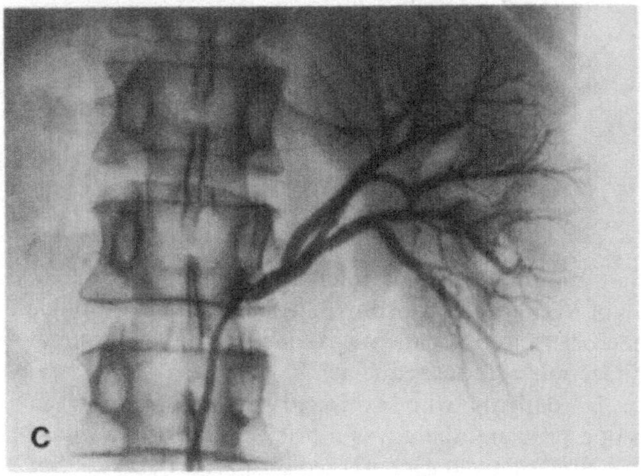

Fig. 8 A–C. Pre- (**A**), post- (**B**), and one-year-post-angioplasty (**C**) arteriograms in a patient with an atherosclerotic stenosis.

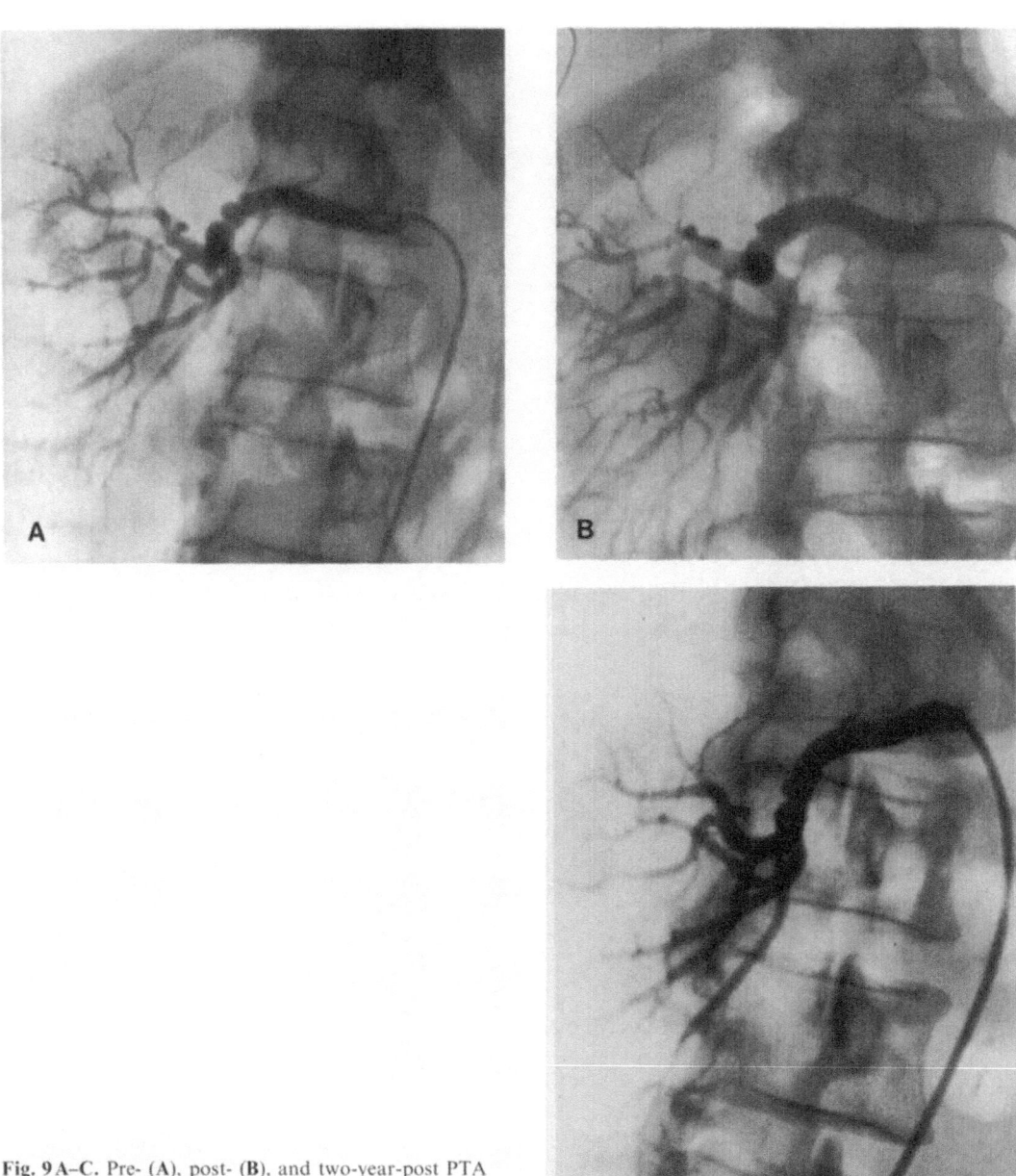

Fig. 9A–C. Pre- (A), post- (B), and two-year-post PTA (C) arteriograms in a patient with fibromuscular dysplasia. There was no gradient present at the time of the two year study.

that required surgical intervention. Three patients, all of whom were in Group 3, developed acute tubular necrosis, and one patient sustained a small subintimal dissection without sequelae.

In patients who exhibited marked changes in blood pressure, there was a brief, initial rise in blood pressure followed by a marked drop. It is believed that this early rise in blood pressure may be the result of rapid renin washout. The low point in blood pres-

sure, which was frequently reached in the two- to six-hour period after angioplasty, frequently required vigorous fluid replacement and, occasionally, vasopressor therapy (Fig. 6).

Discussion

PTRA is a relatively simple procedure that can be performed by an experienced angiographer with little risk to the patient with normal renal function. If it can be shown that PTRA is simpler, safer, and as effective over the long-term as renal artery surgery, revascularization may take the place of the classic operative procedures for the management of renovascular hypertension.

The mortality rate for operations performed for renovascular hypertension varies with reporting centers; the operative mortality reported by the National Cooperative Study was 5.9% [1]. While current series report no operative mortality, the operative morbidity and loss of productive work time that ensue, even under the most favorable circumstances, cannot be ignored. In contrast, PTRA offers a procedure with little morbidity. A short (72-hour) hospital stay with obvious cost-effectiveness is possible provided that PTRA is a one-time event. However, restenosis has not been a rare occurrence; for example, five patients in one series with solitary kidneys who underwent PTRA [11] have gone on to restenosis (M.Y. Yune, personal communication). If a large percentage of recurrent renal artery stenosis develops with PTRA, and repeated PTRAs or operations are required, this savings may be lost. However, the potential for recurrent stenosis after PTRA must be balanced against the graft failure or abnormality rate of approximately 20% and nephrectomy rate of 10% in most surgical series.

Medical management of renovascular hypertension remains a poor alternative. Hunt [2] reported that despite similar blood pressure control, medically managed patients fared much worse than their surgically managed counterparts. At nine years 84% of those operated on were alive as opposed to only 43% of those medically managed (Fig. 7). In addition, the risk of renal artery stenosis progressing to occlusion is not overcome by medical management.

While the dramatic decrease in blood pressure and renin values found in our Group I patients shortly after PTRA and the similar findings of Millan [12] are evidence of PTRA's immediate effectiveness, insufficient time has passed to allow for a long-term comparison of cases treated by PTRA and those managed by an operative approach. It is possible, however, to compare the results for a given time period based on a cure/improvement rate. In Group 1 patients, the results compare favorably with surgical series based on renin activity, especially since most surgical series include relatively large numbers of patients with fibromuscular disease. The 90% rate of cure or improvement in our Group 1 patients at six months compares favorably with the Indiana University Medical Center results of a 90% cure or improvement rate, a 5% failure rate, and a 5% operative

mortality rate in 77 patients, 11 of whom had nephrectomy as their operation [13].

We have had the opportunity to restudy a number of patients electively. Figures 8 and 9 are two-year follow-up arteriograms in patients with, respectively, arteriosclerotic and fibromuscular dysplastic disease. While the angiographic appearance in the patient with fibromuscular dysplasia has deteriorated somewhat, this has not been reflected in any hemodynamic changes.

While the subintimal dissection that occurred in one of our patients was small and did not require surgery, PTRA has a number of inherent risks that can result in serious complications. It is because of this potential for complications that a surgeon experienced in the management of renovascular hypertension must be available within the institution in the event that damage is done to the renal artery and/or kidney during the PTRA procedure. While we have not been able to document any loss of renal tissue, evidence of cholesterol embolization, or renal artery damage, these are potential problems.

Clearly over the short-term, PTRA appears to be at least equal to surgery in the management of renovascular hypertension in terms of patient safety, blood pressure control, and cost-effectiveness. It remains to be seen, however, if PTRA will provide lasting results. The renal artery is subject to high flows (300 ml per minute) and great turbulent stresses in its proximal portion and should provide a stern test for percutaneous transluminal angioplasty procedures.

References

1. Foster, J.H., Maxwell, M.H., Franklin, S.S., Bleifer, K.H., Trippel, O.H., Julian, O.C., De Camp, P.T., Varady, P.T.: Renovascular occlusive disease: Results of operative management. JAMA 231:1043–1048, 1975
2. Hunt, J.C., Strong, C.G.: Renovascular hypertension: Mechanisms, natural history and management. Am. J. Cardiol. 32:562–574, 1973
3. Dotter, C.T., Judkins, M.P.: Transluminal treatment of arteriosclerotic obstruction. Circulation 30:654–670, 1964
4. Grüntzig, A., Bollinger, A., Brunner, U., Schlumpf, M., Wellauer, J.: Perkutane Rekanalisation chronischer arterieller Verschlüsse nach Dotter – eine nicht-operative Kathetertechnik. Schweiz. Med. Wochenschr. 103:825–831, 1973
5. Grüntzig, A., Kuhlmann, U., Vetter, W., Lutolf, U., Meier, B., Siengenthaler, W.: Treatment of renovascular hypertension with percutaneous transluminal dilatation of a renal artery stenosis. Lancet 1:801–802, 1978
6. Grüntzig, A., Kuhlman, U., Vetter, W.: Percutaneous transluminal dilatation of atherosclerotic renal artery stenosis. Circulation 58, Part II, II-213, 1978

7. Grüntzig, A., Kumpe, D.A.: Technique of percutaneous transluminal angioplasty with the Grüntzig balloon catheter. Am. J. Roentgenol. 132:547–552, 1979
8. Couch, N.P., Sullivan, J., Crane, C.: The predictive accuracy of renal vein renin activity in the surgery of renovascular hypertension. Surgery, 79:70–76, 1976
9. Tucker, R.M., Strong, C.G., Brennan, L.A., Sheps, S.G., Brown, R.D., Weinshilbloum, R.M.: Renovascular hypertension: Relationship of surgical curability to renin-angiotensin activity. Mayo Clinic Proc. 53:373–377, 1978
10. Katzen, B., Chang, J., Lukowsky, G., Abramson, E.G.: Percutaneous transluminal angioplasty for treatment of renovascular hypertension. Radiology 131:53–58, 1979
11. Weinberger, M.H., Yune, H.Y., Grim, C.E., Luft, F.C., Klatte, E.C., Donohue, J.P.: Angioplasty for RAS in a solitary functioning kidney. Ann. Intern. Med. 91:684–688, 1979
12. Millan, V.G., Mast, W.E., Ma Dias, N.E.: Nonsurgurical treatment of severe hypertension due to renal artery intimal fibroplasia by PTA. N. Engl. J. Med. 300:1371–73, 1979
13. Lankford, N.S., Donohue, J.P., Grim, C.E., Weinberger, M.H.: Results of surgical treatment of renovascular hypertension. J. Urol. 122:439–441, 1979

Comment

Percutaneous Transluminal Angioplasty of the Renal Artery: A Surgeon's View

David C. Brewster

Department of Surgery, Harvard Medical School, and General Surgical Services, Massachusetts General Hospital, Boston, Massachusetts, USA

Dr. Schwarten's report, describing his personal experience with the treatment of renal artery lesions by percutaneous transluminal renal angioplasty (PTRA), represents an important contribution in this rapidly developing field. In contrast to most prior publications, which have described use of the technique in only one or, perhaps, several patients, the current report is particularly valuable in that it documents experience with a larger series of patients managed over a longer time.

As with any new treatment method, the safety, short-term efficacy, and long-term duration of effect of the procedure must be established by reliable and carefully studied clinical trials. The results must then be compared to those achieved with currently used treatment modalities; in this instance, the results of surgical methods of renal artery reconstruction for revascularization of the ischemic kidney. Surgical experience over the past two decades has been well documented. Currently, a favorable long-term result (implying cure or significant improvement of hypertension) may be anticipated in approximately 90% of properly selected patients undergoing an appropriate surgical procedure performed by an experienced surgeon. Mortality will obviously vary with the type of patient, but should be negligible in the young patient with a fibrodysplastic lesion and not exceed 3–5% in the older patient with lesions typical of generalized arteriosclerosis. Morbidity has been similarly low.

It is fair to say that, in general, surgeons view PTRA with skepticism and concern. Various technical misadventures leading to acute thrombosis of the renal artery or distal embolization of the kidney are clearly potential hazards of PTRA, and it is probably advisable to have a surgeon who is familiar with the patient and his situation available for immediate surgical intervention if necessary. The kidney will not tolerate ischemia secondary to acute arterial occlusion as well as will an extremity, making avoidance of such complications even more important than with iliac or femoral dilatations. Dr. Schwarten's initial success rate of 93%, with only a 5.7% complication rate and no need for emergency surgical intervention, is indeed reassuring in terms of the safety and short-term benefits of the technique. Dr. Schwarten's exact definition of initial success rate is not entirely clear, however. Does this refer simply to successful dilatation of the angiographic lesion or to actual improvement or cure of hypertension?

The current report describes results in terms of average blood pressure responses in various groups of patients. It would be preferable, I believe, to express results in terms of the actual numbers of patients

Address reprint requests to: D.C. Brewster, M.D., General Surgical Services, Massachusetts General Hospital, Fruit Street, Boston, MA 02114, USA

in each group who fell into cured or improved categories, as customarily defined in most prior medical and surgical reports. Nonetheless, the early results suggest that a beneficial response was safely obtained in most patients.

Wide acceptance of PTRA also demands documentation of its long-term duration of effect. This has been well established for surgical procedures, and only time and further experience will establish this aspect of PTRA. Undoubtedly, restenosis will occur, but its incidence has yet to be established. The early experience of Schwarten and others suggests that redilatation may well be feasible and successful, but again this requires further documentation.

It is imperative that further investigation of this potentially valuable technique be carried out as a cooperative effort involving the physician, surgeon, and angiographer. It is important that criteria for patient selection be established, probably similar to those utilized for selection of patients for surgery, and that the procedure not be haphazardly applied to any patient with a renal artery stenosis. Ideally, a randomized trial comparing PTRA and surgery could answer many questions, but may not be feasible in practical terms. Most important, this technique should only be carried out by those experienced with percutaneous transluminal angioplasty in other arterial beds; otherwise I suspect many more kidneys will be lost than hypertensive patients cured.

Comment

Percutaneous Transluminal Angioplasty of the Renal Artery: A Hypertensiologist's View

Eve E. Slater

Hypertension Unit, Department of Medicine, Massachusetts General Hospital and Harvard Medical School, Boston, Massachusetts, USA

Dr. Schwarten's impressive results in the treatment of renovascular disease by percutaneous transluminal renal angioplasty (PTRA) raise high hopes for the future of this technique as a simple, relatively safe, and reasonably inexpensive therapeutic alternative to former therapies that were either less effective for many (medical therapy) or posed a higher risk for some (surgical therapy). Before PTRA becomes widely utilized as an alternative to either therapy, however, we must define its proper indications and critically assess its duration of efficacy. Moreover, certain caveats must be accepted during this phase of data gathering to allow experience with PTRA to accrue while minimizing patient risk.

First, balloon catheter dilation of the renal artery should be attempted only in centers, such as Dr. Schwarten's, that have the requisite expertise in percutaneous angiography and angioplasty of peripheral vascular lesions. Second, angioplasty should be advised only for lesions that appear amenable to this technique since unfavorable lesions are particularly prone to develop complications: certain stenoses are so critical that they do not admit passage of the balloon; others so calcified that they resist dilatation; some so extensive that they extend beyond reach of the balloon; and, occasionally, localized intimal dissection from prior angiography necessitates surgical repair.

Third, certain complications of PTRA must be anticipated with a frequency rate derived from that of percutaneous angiography, viz 5–10%. These complications include, in addition to those encountered by Dr. Schwarten, infection, arterial rupture or dissection, false aneurysm formation, local or retroperitoneal bleeding, subsegmental renal infarction, cholesterol embolization, and balloon rupture with embolization or femoral artery occlusion. While it has been argued that angioplasty is the preferred treatment for patients at high risk from general anesthesia and surgery, it should be cautioned that several of the complications of PTRA require immediate surgical intervention. Thus, PTRA can be performed only in patients without absolute contraindications to surgery and with an experienced vascular surgical team in immediate readiness. The risks of post-PTRA hypotension

Address reprint requests to: E.E. Slater, M.D., Department of Medicine, Massachusetts General Hospital, Fruit Street, Boston, MA 02114, USA

leading to acute tubular necrosis or dye-related renal failure can be minimized by adequate hydration and careful monitoring, as emphasized by Dr. Schwarten.

Lastly, regardless of the indication for PTRA, I still require as a prerequisite the demonstration of increased renin production by the involved side. Despite occasional reports to the contrary, renin production in a concentration higher than that found in the periphery is the most sensitive and accurate predictor of reversibility of renal ischemia. Renin production can be enhanced by the administration of a vasodilator prior to sampling. For further discussion of plasma renin determination, the reader is referred elsewhere [1].

As stated by Dr. Schwarten, there are two general indications for PTRA: correction of renovascular hypertension and preservation of renal function. The decision to recommend angioplasty for either indication, in preference to either definitive surgical repair or medical maintenance, must take into account the specific clinical circumstances. Among patients with unilateral renovascular hypertension of fibromuscular etiology, certain ideal candidates can be identified: first, patients with a major intrarenal stenosis, the surgical repair of which might necessitate sacrifice of renal tissue, and second, younger patients with poorly controlled blood pressure. In these latter patients, definitive surgical repair should be deferred until approximately age 30 or later, since fibromuscular disease is known to progress until the fourth decade.

Among patients with unilateral atherosclerotic renovascular hypertension, the ideal candidate for PTRA is the patient with a relative but not absolute contraindication to surgery, for example, the patient with poorly controlled hypertension and severe angina pectoris or recent myocardial infarction. In these patients, PTRA offers the hope of obviating surgical intervention. Conversely, patients who require extensive revascularization for an associated abdominal aortic aneurysm or aortoiliac disease are ideally treated by surgery.

Patients with bilateral renovascular disease of either atherosclerotic or fibromuscular dysplastic etiol-ogy may represent another special category of patients for whom PTRA is preferable. Traditionally, these patients have been advised to undergo either primary medical therapy or surgery performed in two stages, often with difficulties in blood pressure control encountered during and after the first procedure. The combination of PTRA and surgery or bilateral PTRA performed in sequence has already proven to be most efficacious during short-term follow-up. Among patients with rapidly deteriorating renal function believed due to a renal arterial stenosis, PTRA must be undertaken with caution because of the risk of exacerbating renal dysfunction and only after excess renin production has been demonstrated, thus indicating a degree of reversibility.

Before PTRA is advised for all other patients, the efficacy of the procedure, especially with regard to its duration of effect, must be established through randomized, controlled studies. The argument that PTRA should be attempted as the initial procedure for all patients must be tempered by the knowledge that certain complications of PTRA may require an emergency operation, involving a surgical approach less favorable than that associated with an elective operation. Thus for all such patients, if participation in a randomized study is not feasible, we currently advise a choice of therapy after presenting the alternative pros and cons of each modality.

In sum, PTRA appears to be a safe and effective alternative to medical and surgical therapy of renovascular disease for many patients. Only after judicious application of this modality to carefully selected subsets of patients and critical analysis of the long-term results of this technique will it be possible to appreciate fully the true potential of PTRA in the treatment of renovascular disease.

Reference

1. Slater, E.E., Haber, E.: High blood pressure. In: Scientific American's Medicine – Principles and Progress for Practicing Physicians, edited by E. Rubenstein and D.D. Federman, New York, Scientific American, Inc., 1978, pp. VII-1-31

Percutaneous Dilatation and Recanalization of Iliac and Femoral Arteries

Eberhard Zeitler

Radiodiagnostic Department, Nürnberg Hospitals, Nürnberg, FRG

Abstract. Five-year follow-up studies in patients with superficial femoral arterial occlusions and iliac artery stenoses have demonstrated a high success rate with percutaneous transluminal angioplasty performed by the Dotter technique. The special balloon catheters developed by Grüntzig, a standardized accessory pharmaceutical regimen, and more exact indications have further increased the rate of long-term success; the patency rates now approach 70% after three years. Clinical follow-up studies by Doppler ultrasound are useful for assessing the hemodynamic effects of the procedure.

Key words: Arteries, femoral – Arteries, iliac – Angioplasty – Catheters and catheterization – Interventional radiology.

As a result of technical improvements in the original Dotter [2] catheter, an awareness of the importance of platelet inhibitors, and careful observation of the patient in the first 48 hours after treatment, percutaneous dilatation and recanalization techniques have achieved notable success in the treatment of occlusive disease of the iliac and femoral arteries. Since 1968, we have employed this technique 1,217 times in 1,071 patients. In this paper our experience with percutaneous angioplasty is detailed.

Immediate and Long-Term Results

Catheters

Currently, we use the following types of catheters: (1) bypassing catheters[1] (Zeitler); (2) Teflon dilating catheters in various sizes[1] (Andel); (3) double-lumen catheters[2] (Grüntzig).

In the Aggertalklinik we have had experience with the Dotter technique in its different modifications in 820 patients with 922 recanalizations (Table 1).

This material comprises groups submitted to randomized studies with different drug regimens and different catheters (coaxial dilating set; caged balloon catheter; Fogarty balloon catheter; single Teflon catheter; Grüntzig balloon catheter). After permanent treatment with coumarins, the 6-month patency rate was 25% in patients recanalized with the coaxial dilating set, whereas after recanalization with a single Teflon catheter it was 80%. We have not used the coaxial dilating set since 1974.

In 109 patients with claudication (Stage II) we have now a primary success rate in 96 patients (88%).

Femoral Artery Recanalization

From the overall group of 1,071 patients, follow-up studies over more than five years were carried out in 81 extremities of 79 patients with stage II superficial femoral arterial occlusions treated between December 1968 and November 1971 (Fig. 1). In 21 cases the arteries had been successfully recanalized using 8 French Teflon catheters (today known as bypassing catheters), and 60 cases had been treated with the coaxial dilating set developed by Dotter.

During the follow-up period, 20 patients died. Three legs were amputated (3.7% incidence in seven years) because of gangrene resulting from recurrent occlusion. During the first two years the incidence of restenosis reached 40%. From the third through the fifth year, however, the rate decreased. Of the arteries recanalized, 26% were still patent after five

Address reprint requests to: Prof. Dr. E. Zeitler, Klinikum Nürnberg, Radiologisches Zentrum, Flurstr. 17, D-8500 Nürnberg, Federal Republic of Germany

[1] Cook Europe Aps, DK-2860 Söborg, Denmark
[2] Schneider Medintay, CH-8053 Zürich, Switzerland; Cook Europe Aps, DK-2860 Söborg, Denmark

Table 1. Initial results of recanalization using different modifications of the Dotter technique (820 patients)

Location	No. of procedures	Results[a]			Compli-cations	Additional treatment	
		Success	Partial success	Failure		Operation	Amputation
Iliac stenoses							
single	220	172	32	16	—	1	—
multiple	42	34	4	4	15	—	—
Iliac occlusions	7	1	2	5	—	—	—
Iliac occlusion and iliac stenosis	3	1	2	—	—	—	—
Femoral stenoses							
single	93	78	9	6	—	2	1
multiple	38	32	3	3	9	—	—
Popliteal stenoses	17	11	2	4	8	1	—
Deep artery stenoses	4	4	—	—	—	—	—
Posterior tibial trunc stenoses	1	1	—	—	—	—	—
Deep artery occlusions and deep artery stenoses	1	1	—	—	—	—	—
Femoral artery occlusions (< 10 cm)	304	247	24	33	—	—	—
Femoral artery occlusions (> 10 cm)	133	72	19	42	64	11	1
Popliteal occlusions	34	21	6	7	2	—	—
Other locations[b]	3	2	1	—	—	—	—
Puncture attempts	22	—	—	22			
Total	922	676	104	142	98	15	2

[a] Success = good initial result
Partial success = partial recanalization (residual stenoses)
Failure = unsuccessful recanalization attempt
[b] 2 renal artery stenoses and 1 subclavian artery stenosis

[c] Multiple procedures: 2 locations 36 patients
2 times same location 51 patients
3 times same location 3 patients
5 times same location 1 patient

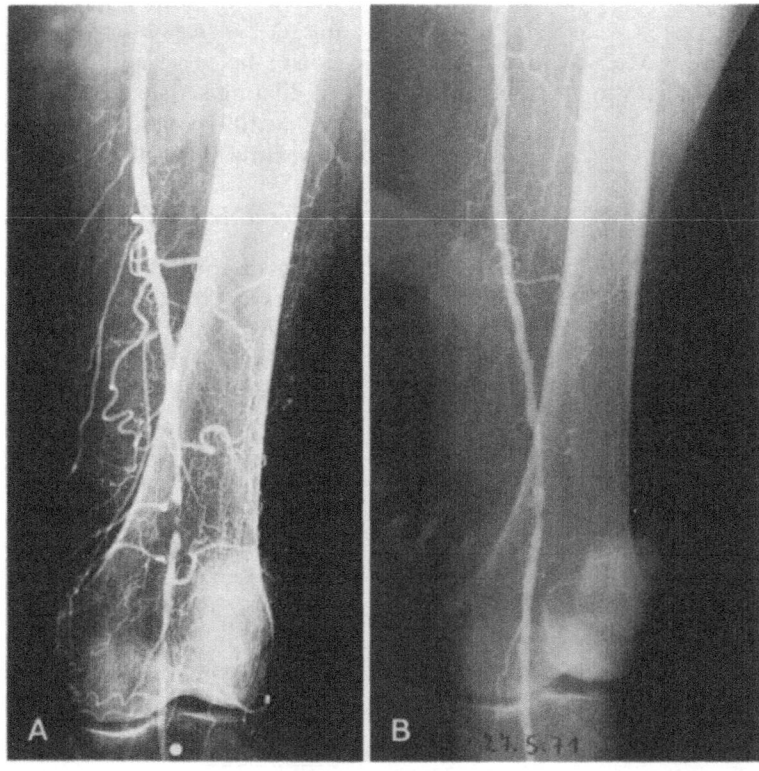

Fig. 1 A and B. Distal femoral artery occlusion 2 cm in length in a 65-year-old man with intermittent claudication due to occlusion of the posterior tibial artery. **A** Angiogram performed in May 1969, before percutaneous angioplasty. The difference between brachial artery and ankle blood pressure was 70 mm Hg. **B** Control angiogram May 1971. The difference in pressure had decreased to 30 mm Hg.

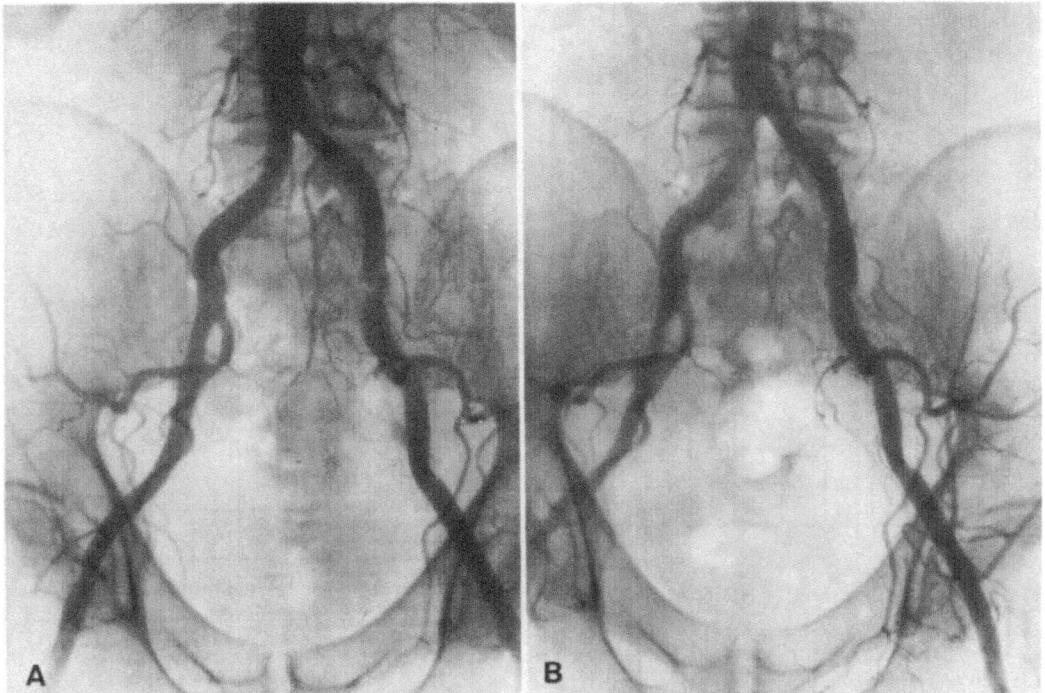

Fig. 2 A and B. A 60-year-old man with stenosis of the left iliac artery and a pressure gradient between the aorta and left common femoral artery of 50 mm Hg. **A** Angiogram before percutaneous angioplasty. **B** Angiogram after percutaneous angioplasty. No pressure gradient was demonstrated.

years, and 20% were patent after six and one-half years.

Previous follow-up examinations of occlusions dilated with the Grüntzig balloon catheter showed a higher patency rate after three years. Continuation of treatment with anticoagulants or platelet aggregation inhibitors has a considerable effect on outcome, however. Our current approach, employing long-term drug administration (see below), has resulted in an increased patency rate.

A cooperative study of 1,184 cases treated in 12 clinics up to March 1977 [5] has now been completed. In this group of patients, one-third of whom had gangrene, the initial success rate with percutaneous angioplasty was 74%, with an early reocclusion rate within two weeks of 11%.

Iliac Artery Recanalization

In the Aggertalklinik, percutaneous transluminal dilatation of iliac artery stenoses (Fig. 2) was performed in 262 iliac arteries (single: 220; multiple: 42). In 78%, the hemodynamic and clinical state was clearly improved. The blood pressure was controlled in each case before and after dilatation of the stenoses. Only dilatations yielding a marked reduction in the blood pressure gradient were considered positive results. A joint study carried out in 12 other clinics showed similar results in 206 additional patients (Fig. 3).

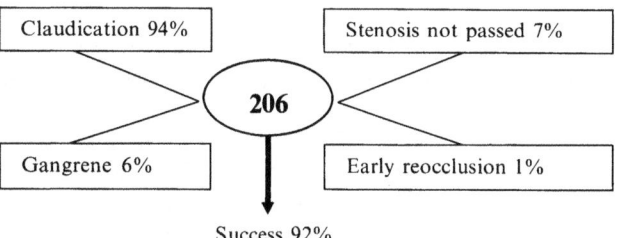

Fig. 3. Percutaneous transluminal dilatation in 12 clinics. Iliac artery stenoses of 206 patients.

Follow-up studies were performed quarterly in 88 patients who had been successfully treated. By 34 months after treatment 16 patients had died. In 69% of the remaining patients the good initial results were still shown three years later, and in 61% they were evident five years later.

Hemodynamic Results

Several studies have shown that percutaneous transluminal angioplasty is associated with an improvement in hemodynamic status. In 1971 we reported a 52% reduction (from 79 to 38 mm Hg) in the blood pressure difference between the brachial and posterior tibial arteries after percutaneous angioplasty in 26 patients [4].

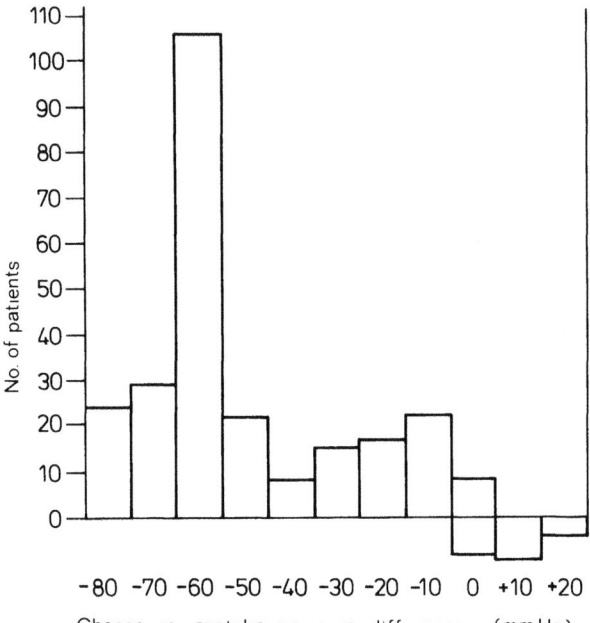

Fig. 4. Change in the systolic pressure difference between the brachial and posterial tibial arteries. Change in pressure from values measured before percutaneous angioplasty and values measured at discharge after percutaneous angioplasty.

Table 2. Percutaneous transcatheter angioplasty in patients with rest pain (Stage III) and gangrene (Stage IV)

Artery	No. of patients	Results[a]		
		Success	Partial success	Failure
Iliac stenoses	13	9 (69%)	2	2
Femoropopliteal stenoses	26	25 (96%)	1	–
Deep femoral artery stenoses	3	3 (100%)	–	–
Femoropopliteal occlusion				
< 10 cm	61	43 (70.5%)	8	10
> 10 cm	29	14 (48%)	2	13
Lower leg artery obliteration	11	6 (54.5%)	1	4
Total	143	100 (70%)	14	29

[a] Success = good initial result
Partial success = partial recanalization (residual stenoses)
Failure = unsuccessful recanalization attempt

Measurement of the systolic pressure difference between the brachial and posterior tibial arteries (Fig. 4) by Doppler ultrasound has shown a reduction in the pressure difference of 55% in successfully recanalized patients and of 45% in all treated patients.

A study by Grüntzig et al. found a 55% reduction in the systolic pressure difference after percutaneous angioplasty of femoral artery occlusions, as compared to a 78% reduction after surgical reconstruction [3].

In 1978, Bollinger [5] demonstrated that after reconstructive surgery in 67 patients the pressure difference between the brachial and posterior tibial arteries decreased from 60 to 7 mm Hg and then increased to 19 mm Hg in 12 months. After percutaneous recanalization in 50 patients the pressure difference decreased from 60 to 19 mm Hg, and 12 months later it was nearly equal the median pressure difference of 20 mm Hg in operated patients. (There were, however, significant differences in Bollinger's group between the operated patients and those who underwent percutaneous treatment.)

Follow-up examinations two and three years later have confirmed these primary hemodynamic improvements. Complete removal of the pressure difference, however, can be expected only in cases in which there are no concomitant occlusions in the lower leg arteries or in which patency can be restored to these arteries also.

Patients with Gangrene

In addition to these encouraging long-term results with the treatment of peripheral vascular disease in patients with claudication, our experiences with angioplasty in patients with gangrene were also successful in the Klinikum in Nürnberg (Table 2).

In this group of 143 patients with rest pain and gangrene there was a notably greater prevalence of women. The mean age of the group was 61 years; the oldest patient was an 87-year old woman. In 60%, clinical diabetes was evident. In none of the cases were all lower leg arteries patent; in 50% only one tibial artery was patent. In 100 cases (70%) we achieved an initial success. Complications requiring surgical intervention occurred in two cases.

Depending on the length of the occluded arterial segment and the outflow, we used either a Teflon bypassing catheter (9 Charrière) or, additionally, one of the Andel's Teflon catheters (9, 10, or 12 Charriere) or a Grüntzig balloon catheter. In cases with poor peripheral outflow it was necessary to work very quickly to avoid prolonged ischemia. Femoropopliteal stenoses were dilated with the Grüntzig catheter after successful passage of the guidewire and the Teflon catheter.

Recanalization was achieved in 70% of the cases with occlusions less than 10 cm in length (Fig. 5) and in 96% of those with femoropopliteal stenoses. In only 8% of those cases in which angioplasty was initially successful was an amputation necessary within three months.

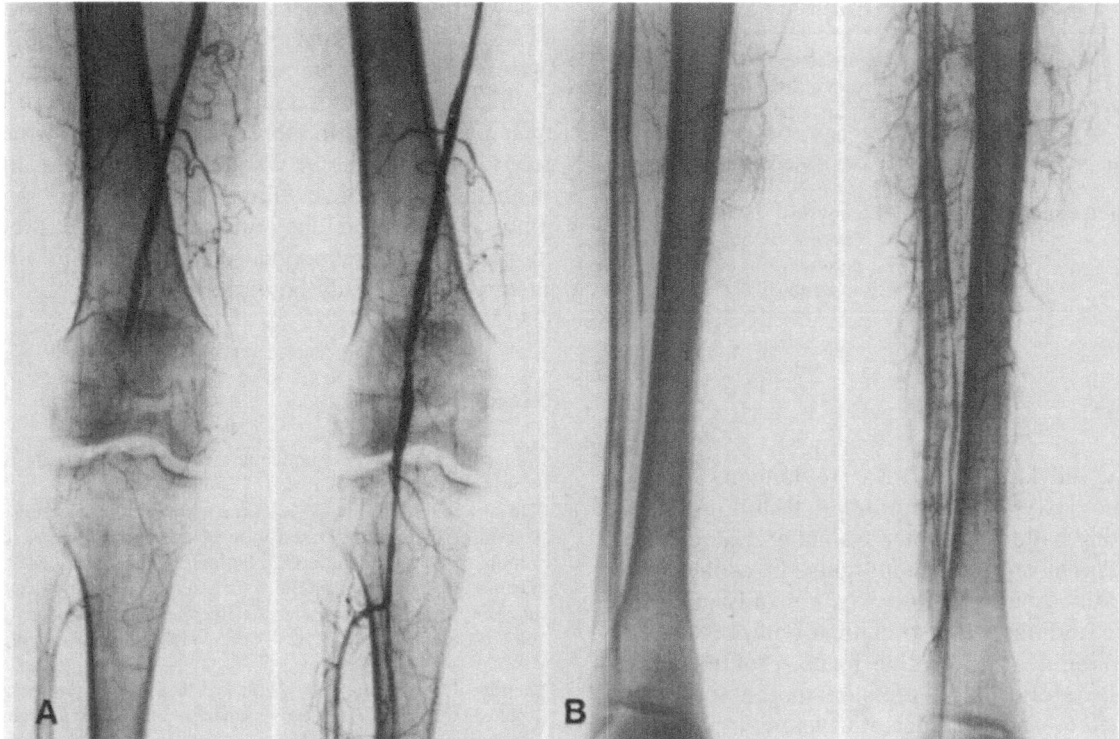

Fig. 5A and B. A 67-year-old woman with diabetes and gangrene of the right foot. **A** Angiography reveals complete occlusion of the popliteal artery, occlusion of the posterior tibial and fibular arteries, and stenosis of the anterior tibial artery. **B** Angiography after recanalization with a single Teflon catheter and dilatation with a balloon catheter, as well as partial dilatation of the stenosis in the anterior tibial artery with a single Teflon catheter. Gangrene was no longer evident after three weeks.

Complications

In a joint study [6] comprising 1,401 patients from four clinics, 35 complications (2.5%) requiring surgical intervention occurred after angioplasty. Thrombotic occlusion, small emboli, and hemorrhage at the puncture site were the most frequent incidents (Table 3). Experience with angioplasty techniques is vital to the avoidance of such complications, while close cooperation between radiologists and surgeons is necessary in the treatment of any complications that may develop.

Pharmaceutical Regimen

We observed that the recanalized femoropopliteal arteries remained patent up to 30 months in 80% in patients given recanalized given whereas the patency rate was only 40% in patients not given anticoagulation therapy. Because only five patients had continued anticoagulation treatment during the subsequent observation period, assessment of the long-term effects of such therapy was impossible. However, in four of the five patients maintained on long-term antico-

Table 3. Joint study of five clinics: Complications in percutaneous angioplasty procedures in 1,401 patients

Complications	No.	%
Hemorrhage	37	2.6
Aneurysm	10	0.7
Perforation	5	0.3
Emboli	47	3.4
Thrombotic occlusion	64	4.6
Requiring surgical treatment	35	2.5

agulant treatment, the femoral artery was patent five years later; in the fifth patient, stenosis did not develop until three years after recanalization.

Because of the findings in our series and in randomized studies, we now use a standardized accessory pharmaceutical treatment (Table 4). For older patients, however, and those with hypertension, gastric ulcers, carcinoma and a history of cerebral infarction, coumarins are contraindicated. In such cases, aggregation inhibitors are probably preferable for long-time treatment. At present, the rate of restenosis is less than 15% in the first year.

Table 4. Accessory pharmaceutical treatment

1. Two days before angioplasty	Acetylsalicylic acid (0.5 g three times a day)
2. After puncture	Intraarterial heparin 5,000 I.U.
3. After angioplasty	Acetylsalicyclic acid for 6–10 days
4. Long-term treatment	Coumarins, starting 2nd or 3rd day after percutaneous angioplasty

Discussion

Both early and late results of percutaneous transluminal angioplasty with the improved techniques using the Grüntzig balloon catheter system and single Teflon catheters have been encouraging. In centers with skilled cardiovascular radiologists, not only good angiographic findings but also clinically impressive improvements and a measurable increase of the mean peripheral systolic blood pressure in the foot have been observed. The incidence of severe complications has been slight.

The major advantage of this method is that it avoids the risks of general anesthesia and operation. Treatment is always carried out under local anesthesia, and the patient's stay in the hospital usually does not exceed three to six days. If stenosis occurs, angioplasty can be repeated. While the chances of success with a bypass operation are unchanged by prior PTA, a thrombendarterectomy has little likelihood of success after percutaneous transluminal angioplasty.

In the interest of the patient, there must be increasing partnership between radiologists and surgeons. In clinics in which percutaneous transluminal angioplasty cannot be offered to patients with localized obliterations in the iliac and femoropopliteal regions, cooperation with experienced radiologists in other departments can easily be organized.

References

1. van Andel, G.J.: Percutaneous transluminal angioplasty. Amsterdam: Excerpta Medica, 1976
2. Dotter, C.T., Judkins, M.P.: Transluminal treatment of arteriosclerotic obstruction. Description of a technic and a preliminary report of its application. Circulation 30:654–670, 1964
3. Grüntzig, A: Die perkutane transluminale Rekanalisation chronischer Arterienverschlüsse mit einer neuen Dilatationstechnik. Baden-Baden, Köln, New York, Verlag Gerhard Witzstrock, 1977
4. Zeitler, E., Schoop, W., Zahnow, W.: The treatment of the occlusive arterial disease by transluminal catheter angioplasty. Radiology 99:19–26, 1971
5. Bollinger, A.: In: Percutaneous Vascular Recanalization: Technique, Applications, Clinical Results, edited by E. Zeitler, A. Grüntzig, W. Schoop. Berlin, Heidelberg, New York, Springer-Verlag, 1978, p. 194
6. Zeitler, E.: In: Percutaneous Vascular Recanalization: Technique, Applications, Clinical Results, edited by E. Zeitler, A. Grüntzig, W. Schoop. Berlin, Heidelberg, New York, Springer-Verlag, 1978, p. 120

Percutaneous Transluminal Angioplasty of Peripheral Vascular Disease: A Two-Year Experience

Ronald F. Colapinto, E. Philip Harries-Jones, and K. Wayne Johnston

Departments of Radiology and Surgery, Toronto General Hospital and University of Toronto, Toronto, Ontario, Canada

Abstract. Over a 23-month period, 172 successful peripheral angioplasties were performed. Life-table analysis gave a two-year patency rate for the total series of 80%. The patency rate for aorto-iliac and femoral-popliteal lesions was 86% and 70%, respectively. Only one late failure occurred in the group of 44 arteries followed for longer than eight months.

Key words: Arteries, femoral – Arteries, iliac – Arteries, popliteal – Arteries, transluminal angioplasty – Catheters and catheterization.

After Dotter introduced the technique of percutaneous dilatation of atherosclerotic stenosis in 1964 [5], the procedure was immediately and enthusiastically adopted in many European centers [13]. At the Toronto General Hospital, however, we did not begin to use this technique until 1978 following the introduction of the Grüntzig balloon catheter [6]. Our initial reluctance was in part due to fear of dislodging atherosclerotic material by the repeated passage of the large catheters used by Dotter and in part due to the lack of reports in English confirming Dotter's results. It is unfortunate, but true, that at our center, like most others in North America, foreign literature tends to be ignored.

Our experience, therefore, differs from that of our European colleagues since many of them used the Dotter technique for up to ten years before the balloon catheter was introduced. The purpose of this paper is to describe our method and the results obtained in the two years since we began the procedure.

Address reprint requests to: R.F. Colapinto, M.D., Department of Radiology, Toronto General Hospital, 101 College Street, Toronto, Ontario M5G 1L7, Canada

Technique

Preliminaries

All patients should be seen in consultation with a vascular surgeon to determine whether surgery, dilatation, or a combination of procedures is indicated. If dilatation is to be performed, it is important that the surgeon be familiar with the patient if he is to offer effective back-up in the event of complications.

A preliminary aortogram or femoral arteriogram is obtained in all cases and should be done as a separate procedure. The interval between arteriogram and dilatation is used to plan the approach to the dilatation, obtain informed consent, and begin premedication. All patients receive 600 mg of aspirin twice a day and 50 mg of persantine every eight hours for two or three days before the dilatation. This medication is also continued for three weeks after a successful dilatation.

Catheter Insertion

Iliac stenoses may be dilated from the contralateral side [1], an approach we initially used for some bilateral iliac lesions. We found, however, that the increased difficulty presented by this approach and the risk of raising an intimal flap in the direction of blood flow far outweighed the inconvenience of a second femoral puncture. We now approach all common and external iliac lesions from the ipsilateral side. The contralateral approach is used only if the stenosis involves the common femoral or internal iliac artery.

The pulseless femoral artery distal to an iliac obstruction can usually be palpated and punctured with little difficulty. If the patient is obese and the femoral artery impalpable, it may be necessary to use fluoroscopy to localize the artery with respect to the femoral head as determined from the previous aortogram.

Distal lesions of the superficial femoral or popliteal arteries require antigrade catheterization of the ipsilateral common femoral artery. This procedure is complicated by the natural tendency of the catheter to enter the profunda femoral artery. This tendency may be prevented by a small curve at the tip of the catheter allowing it to be directed into the superficial femoral artery. Care must be taken to puncture the common femoral artery proximal enough to allow this manoeuvre, especially if the patient is obese.

Catheterization of the Stenosis or Obstruction

The most critical stage of transluminal dilatation is the passage of a wire through the area of stenosis or obstruction before the balloon catheter is inserted. As the approach to a stenotic lesion differs from that employed with a complete obstruction, the methods will be described separately.

Stenosis. To obtain a satisfactory dilatation, it is essential that the catheter stay within the true lumen as it is passed through the stenosis. It is easy to dissect under a plaque if the guidewire is advanced before the catheter. As the guidewire may re-enter the true lumen immediately beyond the plaque, the divergence from the true lumen may not be recognized, even when the catheter is finally advanced over the wire (Fig. 1). Inflation of the balloon within the plaque almost guarantees a bad result. To avoid this, we catheterize the stenosis using a red Kifa catheter with a slight bend at the tip to allow changes in direction. The catheter is advanced slowly through the stenosis under fluoroscopy, using multiple small injections of contrast to determine the direction of the lumen. A straight wire is passed beyond the catheter only if the stenosis is too narrow to allow passage of the catheter alone. In this circumstance, the guidewire adds the stiffness necessary to advance the catheter. The catheter should be advanced only 5–10 mm in this fashion before the guidewire is withdrawn and contrast injected to confirm that it is still within the lumen. J-wires are never used in a stenotic segment as they tend to enter the arterial wall as soon as they emerge from the catheter. It is tempting to use a straight catheter when dealing with a relatively narrow femoral or popliteal artery. Although such a catheter or the wire itself will often pass through the proximal portion of the femoral artery with ease, we still prefer the directional capability of a curved catheter for precise catheterization of the actual stenosis.

Obstruction. A red Kifa catheter, similar to that used for stenosis, is advanced from the common femoral artery to the site of obstruction. As no lumen is present, the probable course of the occluded segment must be determined from the arteriogram. Small injections of contrast into the occluding thrombus may successfully outline the course of the artery by producing a "thrombogram" [3]. Calcification, if present, may also be used as a guide to the direction of the vessel.

The occlusion usually consists of soft, poorly organized thrombus associated with a relatively short primary atheromatous obstruction. The catheter can often be successfully advanced through this thrombus without the aid of the guidewire. The primary atheromatous plaque is almost always situated at the aortic or iliac bifurcation in iliac occlusions and at the adductor foramen in occlusions of the superficial femoral artery. As in stenosis, it may be necessary to use a straight guidewire to pass through this segment before the catheter can be advanced.

Dilatation

Once past the stenosis or obstruction, 5,000 units of heparin are given through the catheter and the Kifa catheter is replaced by a Grüntzig balloon catheter.[1] The appropriate balloon diameter is determined from the previous arteriogram by direct measurement. The balloon chosen should not be wider than the diameter of the vessel immediately adjacent to the diseased area. When choosing the balloon size it should be kept in mind that a relatively small increase in diameter will produce a large increase in blood flow. It is not necessary to restore the vessel to a completely normal angiographic appearance to achieve an excellent clinical result (Fig. 2). We have used a 4-cm-long balloon exclusively, as shorter balloons tend to slip away from the stenosis. Although this may be prevented by leaving the wire in place during the inflation, we prefer to remove the wire to avoid potential thrombus formation and allow perfusion of the vessel through the end hole.

The balloon is inflated for periods of 10 to 15 seconds using dilute contrast medium. Although a pump is available for this purpose, we inflate the balloon manually for more sensitive control of the degree of inflation. Pain, which indicates that the arterial wall is being unduly expanded, should be considered a signal to decrease the degree of inflation.

The immediate success of the procedure is determined by the disappearance of or a decrease in the pressure gradient and an improvement in the appearance of the postdilatation angiogram.

---

[1] Cook Incorporated, Bloomington, Indiana 47401, USA

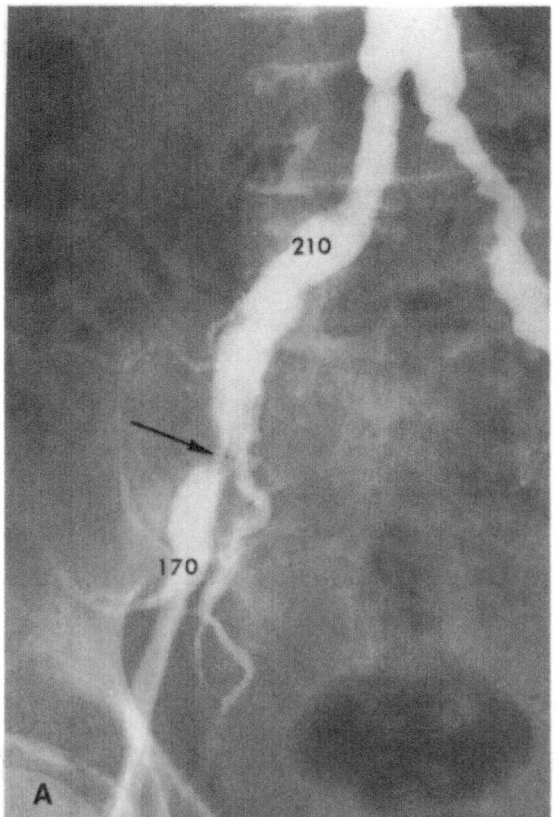

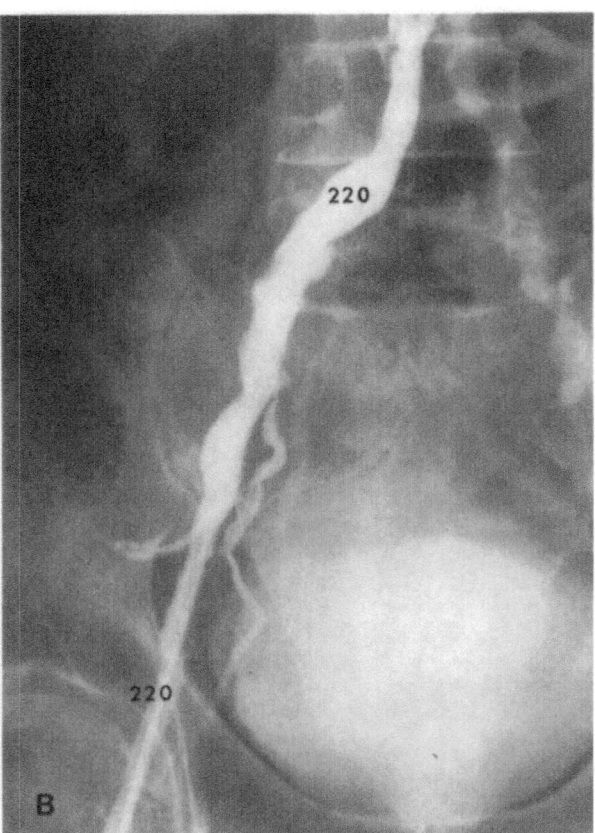

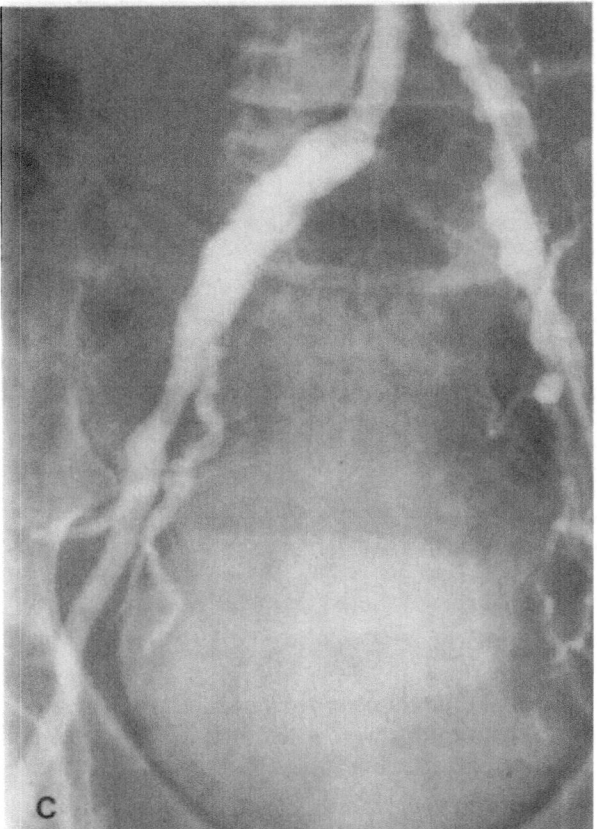

Fig. 1 A–C. A 58-year-old man with severe stenosis of the external iliac artery. The pressure gradient was 40 mm Hg.
A The angiographic catheter has passed through the plaque rather than the true lumen (*arrow*).
B The catheter was withdrawn and following re-catheterization of the true lumen, dilatation was successfully performed, eliminating the pressure gradient.
C Repeat arteriogram five months later shows no evidence of the previous stenosis.

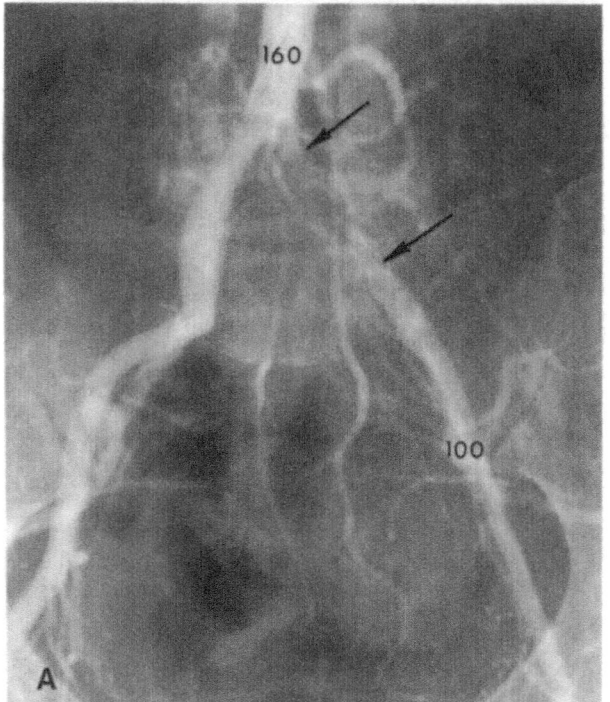

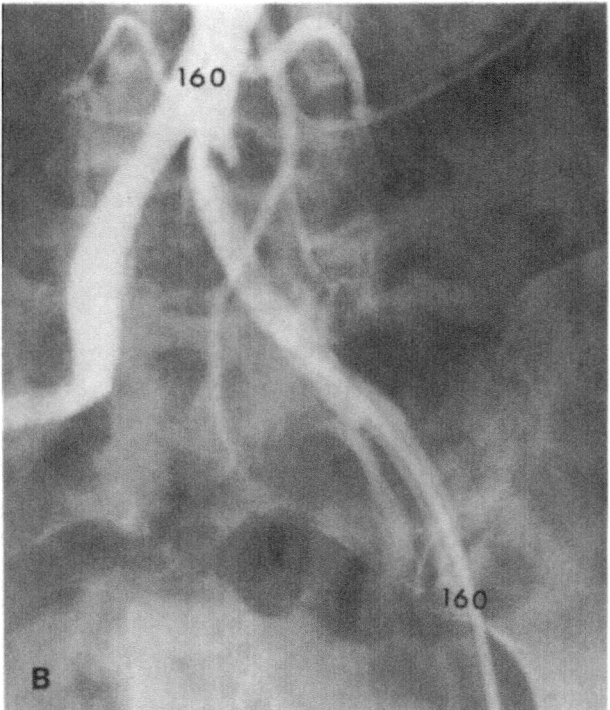

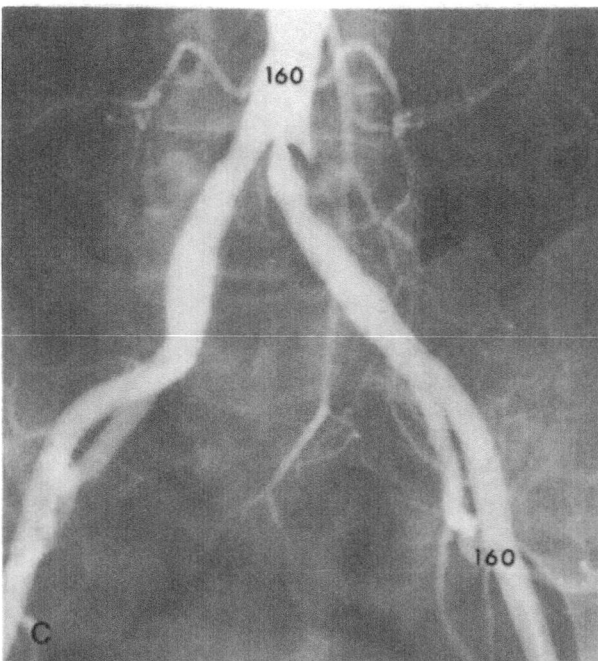

Fig. 2A–C. An active woman of 60 years with severe left buttock pain (aggravated by tennis and dancing).
A There is complete obstruction of the left common iliac artery (*arrows*) with a pressure gradient of 60 mm Hg.
B Immediately following recanalization there is no pressure gradient, and despite the residual proximal narrowing, the patient's symptoms were completely relieved.
C Angiogram obtained 14 months later for right leg claudication caused by a short obstruction of the right superficial femoral artery shows the left common iliac artery unchanged in appearance; no gradient was demonstrated.

Clinical Experience

Transluminal dilatation or recanalization of 193 stenoses or obstructions were attempted in 120 patients over a 23-month period. These figures include each treated lesion. In contrast, our surgical colleagues count only segments (i.e, aorto-iliac and femoral-popliteal) [8]. To avoid confusion, and because we feel that the results of transluminal angioplasty should be assessed on the same basis as the surgical treatment, we have decided to adopt the latter method of tabulation in the future.

We considered the procedure an initial success if there was immediate improvement in the pressure

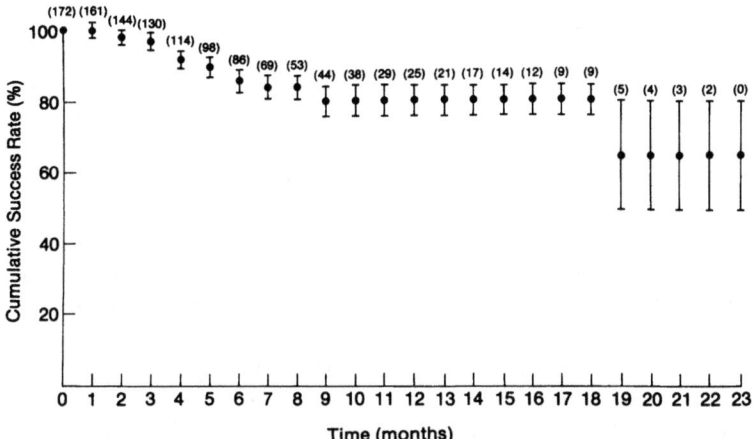

Fig. 3. Life-table analysis of 172 successful dilatations. The cumulative patency rate is shown for each month after the procedure. The vertical bars indicate one standard error from the mean. The number at each point indicates the number of patients still in the series at the beginning of each month. The apparent decrease of the patency rate from 80% to 64% is due to the failure of one iliac dilatation between the 18th and 19th month and is statistically insignificant.

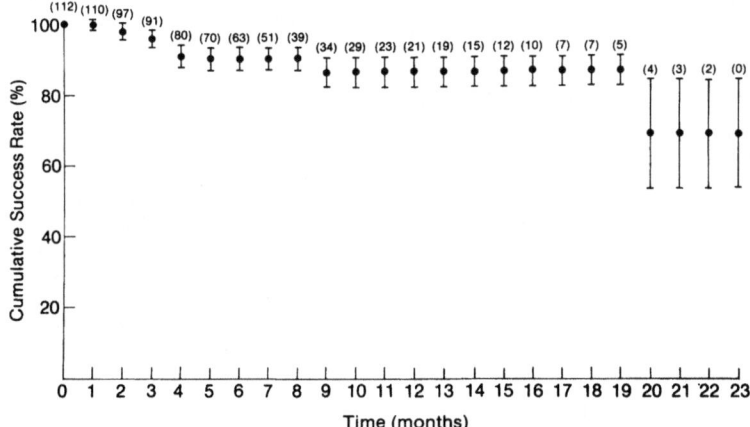

Fig. 4. Life-table analysis of 112 aorto-iliac dilatations gives a cumulative patency rate of 86%.

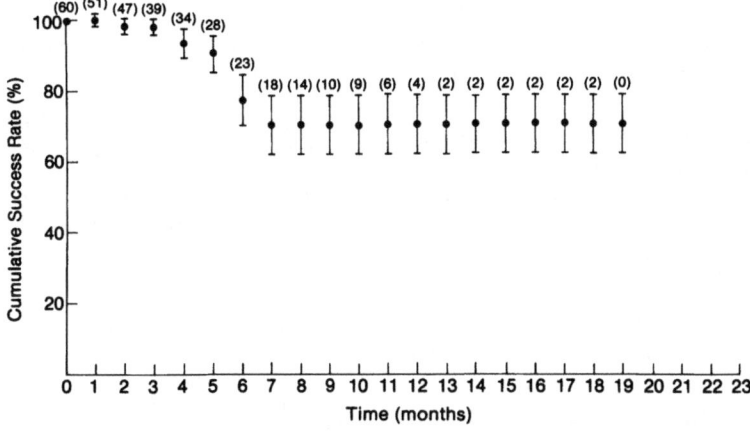

Fig. 5. Life-table analysis of 60 femoral-popliteal dilatations gives a cumulative patency rate of 70%. The longest follow-up in this group is 19 months.

gradient and angiographic appearance. This was accomplished in 172 (89%) of the attempted dilatations. Late results were assessed by clinical status, Doppler flow velocity studies, and ankle-arm pressure ratios. The procedure was not considered a late success unless improvement was noted both symptomatically and by objective measurements.

During the 23-month period, 150 (87.2%) of the 172 successful dilatations remained patent. Life-table analysis of the total series gives a cumulative patency rate of 80% (Fig. 3). The apparent decrease in patency rate at 19 months is due to one failed external iliac stenosis and is statistically insignificant. This failure was the only one to occur in the 44 arteries that were followed for more than eight months. Separate analysis of the iliac and femoral-popliteal lesions for the same period give cumulative patency rates of 86% and 70%, respectively (Figs. 4 and 5).

There were few complications in this series. One patient developed a large groin hematoma that delayed his discharge from the hospital but resolved spontaneously. Thrombosis at the dilatation site occurred in two patients. One thrombosis followed common iliac dilatation and the other dilatation of the profunda femoral artery. In both cases, the thrombosis resolved within two or three hours after heparin administration. There were no clinically significant embolic complications, although small emboli were sometimes noted on post-dilatation angiograms.

Comments

As we expected, the two-year patency rate has increased considerably over the 65% one-year rate previously reported by our group [4]. Although this can be attributed in part to improved technique and greater experience, it also reflects better patient selection, which is one of the most important facets of successful angioplasty [10]. We now avoid long obstructions of the superficial femoral and iliac arteries, although we have had surprising success with total obstruction of either the common or the external iliac arteries (Fig. 2) [3].

Patients with diffuse, multiple stenoses of the iliac or femoral arteries are less likely to receive long-term benefit from dilatation and are probably better treated with bypass surgery. Even these lesions, however, are worth approaching by angioplasty if the patient is not a surgical candidate.

The best results can be expected following dilatation of isolated stenoses of the femoral or iliac arteries. The patency rate is similar to that obtained by surgery, and the low morbidity, low cost, and short hospital stay make dilatation the procedure of choice for these lesions [7, 9, 11]. We have successfully dilat-

ed two distal aortic stenoses, and it appears that these isolated lesions, which tend to occur in women, are also amenable to dilatation [12].

As well as being an alternative to surgery in selected cases, transluminal dilatation is indicated for patients whose disability is not considered severe enough to warrant surgery. Although their symptoms can be controlled by decreased activity, this may involve an unacceptable decrease in the quality of life.

Although the mechanism is still uncertain [2], there is no doubt that transluminal angioplasty works. It is already an established procedure for the treatment of peripheral vascular disease in Europe and inevitably will be accepted in North America.

Acknowledgements. The authors which to acknowledge the assistance provided by Mrs. B. Hanson and Mrs. S. Ungaro in performing the vascular laboratory studies and helping with the follow-up.

References

1. Bachman, D.M., Casarella, W.J., Sos, T.A.: Percutaneous iliofemoral angioplasty via the contralateral femoral artery. Radiology 130:617–621, 1979
2. Castaneda-Zuniga, W.R., Formanek, A., Tadavarty, M., Vlodaver, Z., Edwards, J.E., Zollikofer, C., Amplatz, K.: The mechanism of balloon angioplasty. Radiology 135:565–571, 1980
3. Colapinto, R.F., Harries-Jones, E.P., Johnston, K.W.: Percutaneous transluminal recanalization of complete iliac artery occlusions. Arch. Surg. (in press)
4. Colapinto, R.F., Harries-Jones, E.P., Johnson, K.W.: Percutaneous transluminal dilatation and recanalization in the treatment of peripheral vascular disease. Radiology 135:583–587, 1980
5. Dotter, C.T., Judkins, M.P.: Transluminal treatment of arteriosclerotic obstruction: Description of a preliminary report of its application. Circulation 30:654–670, 1964
6. Grüntzig, A.: Die perkutane Rekanalisation chronischer arterieller Verschlüsse (Dotter-Prinzip) mit einem neuen doppellumigen Dilatationskatheter. Fortschr. Röntgenstr. 124:80–86, 1976
7. Grüntzig, A., Kumpe, D.A.: Technique of percutaneous angioplasty with the Grüntzig balloon catheter. Am. J. Roentgenol. 132:547–552, 1979
8. Johnston, K.W., Colapinto, R.F., Harries-Jones, E.P., deMorais, D., Kalman, P.G., Baird, R.J., Goldman, B.S., Key, J.A., Weisel, R.D.: Results of transluminal dilatation (TLD) in the treatment of peripheral arterial occlusive disease. Can. J. Surg. (in press)
9. Katzen, B.T., Chang, J.: Percutaneous transluminal angioplasty with the Grüntzig balloon catheter. Radiology 130:623–626, 1979
10. Motarjeme, A., Keifer, J.W., Zuska, A.J.: Percutaneous transluminal angioplasty and case selection. Radiology 135:573–581, 1980
11. van Andel, G.J.: Transluminal iliac angioplasty: Long-term results. Radiology 135:607–611, 1980
12. Velasquez, G., Castaneda-Zuniga, W., Formanek, A., Zollikofer, C., Barreto, A., Nicoloff, D., Amplatz, K., Sullivan, A.: Nonsurgical aortoplasty in Leriche syndrome. Radiology 134:359–360, 1980
13. Zeitler, E., Grüntzig, A., Schoop, W., editors: Percutaneous Vascular Recanalization. Technique, Application, Clinical Results. Berlin, Heidelberg, New York, Springer-Verlag, 1978

Percutaneous Transluminal Angioplasty: A Surgeon's View

Nathan P. Couch

Department of Surgery, Harvard Medical School, Brigham and Women's Hospital, Boston, Massachusetts, USA

Key words: Arteries, femoral – Arteries, iliac – Coronary arteries – Angioplasty – Catheters and catheterization – Interventional radiology.

How can surgeons and radiologists collaborate most effectively in furthering percutaneous transluminal angioplasty (PTA)?

Surgeons serve as referral sources, as co-workers in the care of patients requiring both surgery and PTA, and, occasionally, as urgent consultants in acute complications. In a broader way, surgeons can serve as advisers to radiologists in longitudinal observation and reporting of results. In a most important and specific way, surgeons inevitably will contribute to the decision for PTA itself.

The symptomatic indications for PTA or a surgical procedure are quite similar, i.e., disabling claudication or impending gangrene. The choice between the two procedures is based on anatomic considerations as well as on the degree of mortal risk associated with the procedure. Surgery is indicated in long, total occlusions, especially in small caliber arteries, because bypass grafts afford excellent results in such cases. In contrast, short stenoses in large caliber, accessible arteries are an indication for PTA. For example, iliac arterial stenoses are already yielding well to PTA, at least in the early phase (Table), and promising early results are also being reported for the coronary arteries [6, 7]. For the same anatomic reasons, renal artery stenoses offer an especially impor-

tant opportunity for PTA. These lesions can occasionally be troublesome for the surgeon, especially if there are multiple branch occlusions or previous dissection. Beyond this anatomic factor, many patients with atherosclerotic renal artery stenosis are poor surgical risks. For similar reasons, celiac or mesenteric arterial occlusions are also promising for PTA because they too are usually within easy reach of the catheter and often occur in poor-risk patients.

Still another anatomic factor that weighs towards the choice of PTA is infection near the site where the surgical incision would be made, especially if a plastic graft must be used. Under these circumstances, infection of the graft would convert a preoperative threat to a limb into a postoperative threat to life because of the potential disruption of the suture line. For the reasons above, and for others yet to be encountered, surgeons will be ever more inclined to seek help from interventional radiologists as PTA methods reach maturity.

The expected complications of PTA are usually, but not always, surgically manageable, including the most dangerous: arterial rupture and hemorrhage and acute occlusion of a coronary artery. Such events are quite unwelcome in x-ray departments, but disastrous end-results should be minimized by reserving an operating room and a surgical team until the critical PTA maneuvers have been completed.

What are the comparative results so far of PTA and surgery? It is unfortunate that most papers on PTA make little or no reference to surgical reconstruction in similar cases and that almost every author presents data differently. In the Table are summarized the PTA and surgical results for both iliac and femoral obstructions. It is clear that the surgical results are superior in these admittedly heterogeneous groups, but adequate numbers of late results for PTA have yet to be reported, even for that most promising group, the short iliac stenoses. Perhaps this deficiency

Supported in part by the Brigham Surgical Group Foundation

Address reprint requests to: N.P. Couch, M.D., Department of Surgery, Brigham and Women's Hospital, 75 Francis Street, Boston, MA 02115, USA

Table

Artery and procedure	No. pts.	Mortality (%)	Serious complications	Initial success (%)	Late patency (%)	
					3 yr.	5 yr.
Iliac						
PTA [4, 5, 12]	392	N.S.; 1%	3–4	76–92	N.S.	N.S.
Surgery [1, 9]	1,090	2–3	N.S.	96–99	90	82–95
Femoral-popliteal						
PTA [5, 11, 13, 14]	2,804	N.S.	6–20	70–76	N.S., 15–30	N.S., 10–30
Surgery [8, 9]	880	1–4	N.S.	76–98	60–77	57–78

N.S. = Not stated

will be remedied in the next two or three years with later and more extensive publications.

A few points about general policy should be made. Any department of radiology will profit from concentrating PTA experience in the hands of only two or three radiologists. As in any other clinical endeavor, it is a poor idea for a large number of people to become occasional operatives. All effort should be focused on producing the best possible results and this can only be achieved by very experienced workers. While PTA itself is a seemingly straightforward technical exercise, the indications for and implications of the procedure can be complex, and PTA therefore deserves great attention to detail and the benefits of experience.

With reference to informed consent, patients should be told that these procedures are exploratory, and radiologists beginning to perform them should tell their patients that experience is limited. In the end, this candid approach will yield large benefits in terms of the good will of referring physicians and their patients.

It is important for the radiologist to see the patient, not only on the first post-PTA day, but also over the long term. Surgeons' cooperation will always be helpful in this follow-up.

In addition to the standard clinical criteria, the Doppler ultrasound technique might be used by radiologists to quantify their late results. This method, which is well known to all surgeons, would provide a simple, noninvasive way to document ankle pressure changes before and after dilatation. It is especially informative when post-exercise testing is carried out.

Finally, there are a few general lessons that surgeons have learned from performing similarly new procedures. Interventional radiologists might establish a central registry similar to that maintained by the Transplant Groups since 1964. Somebody, somewhere, should monitor PTA activities, should be available for advice, and should give radiologists the

feeling that there is central support to stimulate the best possible performance. The program would merely require modest financing and the direction by one of the premier radiologic societies. A universal protocol sheet will be essential because details of technique are just as important as they are in any other arteriographic or surgical procedure. When results are reviewed and differences in those results appear, interventional radiologists will need to know all of the determinant details.

In closing, I encourage all radiologists interested in PTA to proceed with patience, care, and optimism. They will surely make important contributions. In concert, surgeons will render progressively more support as they see how radiologists can help their patients and themselves.

References

1. Brewster, D.C., Darling, R.C.: Optimal methods of aortoiliac reconstruction. Surgery 84:739–748, 1978
2. Darling, R.C., Linton, R.R., Razzuk, M.A.: Saphenous vein bypass grafts for femoropopliteal occlusive disease. Surgery 61:31–40, 1967
3. Deweese, J., Rob, C.G.: Autogenous venous bypass grafts five years later. Ann. Surg. 174:346–356, 1971
4. Dotter, C.T., Rosch, J. Anderson, J.M., Antonovic, R., Robinson, M.: Transluminal iliac arterial dilatation nonsurgical catheter treatment of atheromatous narrowing. JAMA 230:117–124, 1974
5. Grüntzig, A., Zeitler, E.: Cooperative study of results of PTR in twelve different clinics. In: Percutaneous Vascular Recanalization: Technique, Application, Clinical Results, edited by E. Zeitler, A. Grüntzig, W. Schoop. Berlin, Heidelberg, New York, Springer-Verlag, 1978
6. Grüntzig, A.R., Senning, A., Siegenthaler, W.E.: Nonoperative dilatation of coronary artery stenosis. N. Engl. J. Med. 301:61–68, 1979
7. Grüntzig, A., Myler, R., Stertzer, S.: Percutaneous transluminal coronary angioplasty (PTCA): Present state of the art (abstract). Circulation 60:264, 1979

8. Maini, B.S., Mannick, J.A.: Effect of arterial reconstruction on limb salvage. Arch. Surg. 113:1297–1304, 1978
9. Malone, J.M., Moore, W.S., Goldstone, J.: The natural history of bilateral aortofemoral bypass grafts for ischemia of the lower extremities. Arch. Surg. 110:1300–1306, 1975
10. Reichle, F.A., Rankin, K.P., Tyson, R.R., Finestone, A.J., Shuman, C.: Long-term results of 474 arterial reconstructions for severely ischemic limbs: A fourteen year follow-up. Surgery 85:93–100, 1979
11. Schmidtke, I., Zeitler, E., Schoop, W.: Late results of percutaneous catheter treatment (Dotter's technique) in occlusion of the femoro-popliteal arteries. In: Percutaneous Vascular Recanlization: Technique, Application, Clinical Results, edited by

E. Zeitler, A. Grüntzig, W. Schoop. Berlin, Heidelberg, New York, Springer-Verlag, 1978
12. Schoop, W., Levy, H., Cappius, G., Mansjoer, H., Zeitler, E.. Early and late results of PTD in iliac stenosis. In: Percutaneous Transluminal Angioplasty: Technique, Application, Clinical Results, edited by E. Zeitler, A. Grüntzig, W. Schoop. Berlin, Heidelberg, New York, Springer-Verlag, 1978
13. Wierny, L., Plass, R., Portsmann, W., Long-term results in 100 consecutive patients treated with transluminal angioplasty. Radiology 112:543–548, 1974
14. Zeitler, E., Schoop, W., Zahnow, W.: The treatment of occlusive arterial disease by transluminal catheter angioplasty. Radiology 99:19–26, 1971

Comment

Percutaneous Transluminal Angioplasty: Cooperation among Specialties

Eberhard Zeitler

Radiodiagnostic Department, Nürnberg Hospitals, Nürnberg, FRG

It is appropriate that a well-known vascular surgeon should encourage cardiovascular radiologists interested in percutaneous transluminal angioplasty (PTA) to proceed with patience, care, and optimism. These counsels are worth heeding by all who are concerned with PTA, and I wish to thank Dr. Couch for his encouraging contribution.

I would also like, however, to comment on some points raised by Dr. Couch's remarks.

1. A standby surgical team for immediate intervention in the case of PTA complications is only necessary during dilatation of coronary artery stenoses. Arterial ruptures with hemorrhage requiring emergency surgical care usually do not occur during dilatation of renal, pelvic, and leg arteries.

2. Radiologists carrying out PTA must (a) be familiar with all problems of occlusive vascular disease; (b) be able to carry out the necessary medical treatment, including the prescription of appropriate

medications; and (c) be capable of performing follow-up studies effectively.

It is, therefore, true that only a few individuals in each institution who have had thorough training should perform this technique.

3. Follow-up controls using Doppler ultrasound only deliver comparable information if the difference or the quotient is determined between the mediam systolic blood pressure at the brachial artery and at the ankle.

4. Cooperation between the cardiovascular radiologist and clinician must also extend to the vascular surgeon and the angiologist, both of whom should be included in discussions on the indications for the procedure as well as in carrying out follow-up treatment and studies. Objective assessment by Doppler ultrasound of the results of long-term, follow-up treatment can best be carried out by the angiologist or clinical physiologist.

Finally, I wish to mention that interested colleagues may obtain the draft of a uniform protocol for PTA studies from me, upon request. Moreover, it is also possible to join a cooperative study.

Address reprint requests to: Prof. Dr. E. Zeitler, Klinikum Nürnberg, Radiologisches Zentrum, Flurstr. 17, D-8500 Nürnberg, Federal Republic of Germany

Transcatheter Vessel Occlusion: Selection of Methods and Materials

Alan J. Greenfield

Department of Radiology, Harvard Medical School and Massachusetts General Hospital, Boston, Massachusetts, USA

Abstract. Transcatheter vessel occlusion (TCVO) is increasingly used for control of hemorrhage, palliative and preoperative tumor embolization, organ function ablation, and obliteration of arteriovenous fistulae and malformations. Methods for TCVO include transcather electrocoagulation, "staining" with contrast, the use of balloon-tipped catheters, and embolization. The choice of method and material depends on whether proximal occlusion of feeding vessels or arteriocapillary occlusion is desired, the vascular anatomy of the lesion, the safety with which the lesion can be embolized, and the type of lesion being treated.

Embolization is the most frequently employed modality. Available materials include autologous tissue, absorbable hemostatics, synthetic particulates, and liquid polymers. Each material has advantages and disadvantages that make it desirable in certain situations and less useful in others. Complications of TCVO may be disastrous, but can be avoided with careful attention to detail. The specific features of the lesion determine the choice of materials and techniques.

Key words: Gelfoam – Embolism, therapeutic – Catheters and catheterization – Interventional radiology.

Transcatheter vessel occlusion (TCVO), which was first introduced in the 1930s for the treatment of carotid-cavernous fistulae, has been widely used in the management of hemorrhage, the palliative and preoperative management of tumors and arteriovenous malformations, organ function ablation, and occlusion of arteriovenous fistulae [1]. Various methods and materials (ranging from autologous tissue to plas-

tic polymers) may be employed for TCVO, and there is controversy over the most appropriate for a given indication. In this paper an attempt is made to set criteria for a rational approach to the selection of such methods and materials. These criteria will be based on evaluation of the following issues:

1. Whether occlusion should be aimed at the arteriolar or capillary level or oriented to the proximal occlusion of larger vessels.
2. How the vascular anatomy of the lesion or the target organ affects the choice of materials.
3. How reflux and occlusion of non target vessels can be prevented.
4. How future treatment plans affect the choice of materials.
5. Complications specific to various lesions and their prevention.

Methods

Methods currently applied for transcatheter vessel occlusion include: electrocoagulation, "staining," the use of balloon-tipped catheters, and embolization.

With transcatheter electrocoagulation, which is discussed elsewhere in this issue, some notable successes have been reported, although the method has not been widely applied clinically [2]. Staining of lesions using contrast media and/or toxic therapeutic agents [3], which is functionally similar to embolization, will not be discussed here.

Catheters with permanently attached balloons near their tips permit temporary, reversible occlusion of relatively large vessels; they are also useful for the prevention of reflux of embolic material during embolization with particulate matter [4]. Balloon catheters of the Wholey or Meditech variety are similar to standard angiographic catheters; the Fogarty

Address reprint requests to: R.I. White. Jr., M.D., Department of Radiology, Johns Hopkins Hospital. Baltimore, MD 21205, USA
ton, MA 02114, USA

or Swan-Ganz balloon catheters are polyvinyl chloride and cannot be used for selective catheterization of vessels. However, small (2 French) Fogarty catheters can be introduced through catheterization used for catheters. Any of these catheters may be life-saving when used for temporary control of massive hemorrhage to stabilize the patient prior to an operation [5]. If the anatomy is suitable, more prolonged vascular occlusion may be accomplished by the balloon occlusion of feeding vessels, since the consequent thrombosis of vessels distal to the balloon catheter permits subsequent removal of the balloon [6].

Because embolization of vessels via the angiographic catheter is currently the most frequently employed TCVO method, the various embolic materials will be dealt with in more detail.

Available Embolic Materials

The table lists various materials available for transcatheter embolization. There are many ways to divide these materials into groups, including liquid vs. solid, absorbable vs. nonabsorbable, vessel size occluded, clinical vs. research availability, and tissue reactivity. The table is organized according to permanence of occlusion, and within that organization, is subdivided by the physical characteristics of the material; availability for clinical use is indicated [7–12].

Autologous Materials. Early attempts at embolic control of arteriovenous fistulae were carried out using autologous clot, muscle, fat, fascia lata, or dura [13]. The first attempts at control of gastrointestinal and pelvic hemorrhage were also performed with autologous clot [2, 14]. Readily available, easily prepared and intrinsically sterile, autologous clot suffers rapid dissolution, even when modified with aminocaproic acid, and also has a propensity to fragment, leading to somewhat unpredictable distribution. Because of the availability of the absorbable hemostatic agents described below, there is little indication for the use of autologous clot in current angiographic practice. One might, however, consider it when life-threatening hemorrhage necessitates intervention, reflux of embolic material is inevitable because of the position of the catheter tip, and rapid dissolution of material which may reflux is desirable.

Absorbable Hemostatics. Absorbable gelatin sponge (Gelfoam), currently the most popular material for embolization, is widely available, sterile, easy to tailor to the size of vessel to be occluded, and almost ideal in being absorbed in a period of days. It suffers from lack of radiopacity. It is easy to handle and simple

Table. Materials available for transcatheter embolization

Materials	Recanalization	Reactivity
Autologous		
*Clot		
Native	6–12 hours	None
Modified	12–24 hours	None
*Tissue		
Muscle	Longterm	Moderate
Dura		
Fascialata		
Absorbable particulate		
*Surgical gelatin		
(Gelfoam)	Days	Moderate
*Oxidized cellulose		
(Oxycel)	Days	
*Microfibrillar collagen		
(Avitene)	Days-weeks	
Nonabsorbable particulate		
*Polyvinyl alcohol		
(PVA)	Permanent	Low
*Silicone spheres	Permanent	None
Bristle brushes	Permanent	None
*Steel coils	Permanent	Variable
*Detachable balloons	Permanent	Low
Polystyrene spheres	Permanent	None
Polymers		
Isobutyl 2-cyanoacrylate		
(IBC)	Permanent	Controversial
Silicone rubber	Permanent	Low
Polyurethane	Permanent	Severe

*   Available for clinical use

to introduce through angiographic catheters as small as 0.025-inch inner diameter. Other materials such as oxidized cellulose (Oxycel) and microcrystalline collagen (Avitene) are also available, but because they are more difficult to handle and offer no advantage over Gelfoam, they have not achieved widespread acceptance [7, 12]. Gelfoam is also available as a powder with properties similar to those of Avitene. Both these materials, as fine powders, produce occlusion at the arteriolar level and may lead to severe tissue ischemia [12]. While this is desirable when dealing with tumors, it is a drawback when there is reflux into normal tissue or when the powder passes through lesions with arteriovenous shunting resulting in subsequent microembolization into the pulmonary circulation. There would appear to be little advantage to Avitene over Gelfoam and much to recommend against its use.

In our practice, Gelfoam is the material of choice when non-permanent vascular occlusion is desired and safe Gelfoam is the of the target vessel can be achieved with catheters large enough to allow introduction of particles of appropriate size. Attention to aseptic technique is particularly important when Gelfoam is used, as bacteriologic analysis of wetted Gelfoam shows rapid contamination of the material when left exposed even in a sterile procedure room (M. Wholey, unpublished data). It is also noteworthy that large particles of Gelfoam introduced through standard angiographic catheters fragment into pieces of much smaller size as they are forced through the catheter tip and the stopcock [4].

Nonabsorbable Microparticles. The most important material in this group is polyvinyl alcohol sponge (Ivalon) (PVA). Microspheres of various types, including silicone rubber, polystyrene, and methyl methacrylate, have also been proposed, but because of difficulties in handling and introducing these materials, we rarely use them. Ivalon is attractive because it is similar to Gelfoam in its handling properties and occluding effect but produces permanent occlusions with minimal tissue reactivity [11]. It is somewhat cumbersome to prepare and sterilize, which is a minor disadvantage. As it is compressible but reexpands considerably in all dimensions on exposure to a liquid environment, occlusion of relatively large vessels through relatively small lumen catheters is possible. We use Ivalon for palliative embolization of tumors and arteriovenous malformations but rarely for control of hemorrhage.

Nonabsorbable Macroparticulate Materials. Most important in this group are steel coil devices [15] and detachable balloons [16–18]. Other materials, such as spheres made of silicone rubber or other plastics and bristle brushes [19], are cumbersome to use and have little to recommend them. The important characteristic of this class of devices is that they are used to occlude relatively large vessels with an end result similar to surgical ligation. Thus, they ordinarily are not used alone when control of active hemorrhage and tumor or organ infarction is desired. However, they are ideal for control of arteriovenous fistulae, occlusion of feeding vessels to a lesion following more peripheral embolization with Gelfoam, or occlusion of relatively large vascular lacerations. The coil device is available in a large size with a diameter of 5 mm after introduction, and it does not requires a tapered catheter for introduction. A smaller version, of approximately 4 mm diameter after introduction, is also available; it will pass safely through a 5 French offer after polyethylene catheter, making this system more flexible.

The detachable miniballoons, which are available for occlusion of vessels up to 4 mm in diameter, offer two advantages over the steel coil device which offset

their expense and somewhat cumbersome introduction system [17]. They may be retrieved so that vessel occlusion may be tested before permanent detachment of the balloon, and they are flow directed so that they may be injected at a considerable distance from a lesion and yet be directed to the lesion by blood flow. For applications such as in arteriovenous fistulae and where reflux of particulate emboli is potentially disastrous, these materials are ideal. Miniballoons are rendered radiopaque by the use of contrast for inflation.

Liquid Polymers. Liquid plastic polymers are introduced in the liquid or semi-solid state and undergo polymerization, either due to the effects of a catalyst premixed with the liquid material, or on contact with blood (or other ionized material). None of these materials are approved for clinical use except on an investigational basis, and considerable experience is required in their use. The most commonly known material is isobutyl 2-cyanoacrylate (IBC), a highly refined version of instant bonding glue available commercially for home use in mending plastics and metals [20]. This material remains liquid until it comes in contact with ionized materials, at which time it polymerizes almost instantly. It can be rendered radiopaque by mixing it with nonionized contrast media such as Pantopaque or Ethiodol or with powdered tantalum. It bonds rapidly to tissue and must be handled carefully to avoid damage to eyes and skin. It is useful in TCVO because it can be introduced through small diameter catheters and yet will occlude vessels of large diameter. It may be used to provide either proximal occlusion or "casting" of lesions. Its tissue reactivity has been controversial, with animal studies suggesting a considerable inflammatory response [8]. However, histologic specimens from patients have shown little or no evidence of reactivity [21]. We have found the material particularly useful in two situations: (1) when the rent in a vessel is so large that particulate material of sufficient size cannot be introduced with standard catheters, and (2) when catheterization of the vessel can only be achieved through a coaxial system.

Other liquid polymers based on silicone rubber and polyurethane have been used for transcatheter embolization [22, 23]. They are more viscous than IBC and larger catheters are necessary. The silicone rubber preparation is ideal for the obliteration of large arteriovenous malformations because of its ability to form a cast of the lesion's vascular tree. The polyurethane material, which is less viscous and so easier to handle, causes local tissue toxicity, and, therefore, its use is limited to experimental applications at this time.

Complications of Embolization

Complications of TCVO may be divided in two major categories: those related to ischemia induced by embolization and those due to reflux of occluding materials with occlusion of vessels outside the target area. These complications can be eliminated or their effects greatly reduced by careful attention to detail.

In our experience, the most common side effect related to tissue ischemia is pain. The degree of pain varies from tissue to tissue, and it can be severe, requiring intravenous narcotic administration for several days. A more important side effect related to tissue ischemia is sepsis with abscess formation, which has been reported both in the spleen and the liver [24], while gas formation without evidence of bacterial infection has been reported in the kidney [25]. It is not clear in these cases whether bacteria were introduced with the embolic material or whether superinfection occurred as a result of bacteremia from indwelling catheters, concomitant infections, or surgical manipulations. Introduction of sepsis with the embolic material can be completely eliminated when careful attention is paid to aseptic technique, meticulous skin preparation, careful handling of embolic materials, and, especially whencareful attention is gans, the use of antibiotic coverage [26].

Emboli may pass through a large arteriovenous communication and reach the lungs [27] unless care is taken to use embolic material of appropriate size. Reflux of embolic material has produced cerebral, spinal cord, renal, and bowel infarction, as well as occlusion of an extremity vessel. The conditions under which reflux occurs and methods for its prevention have been studied experimentally [4]. Preventive measures include:

1. Balloon occlusion of the embolized vessel
2. Superselection of the vessel to be catheterized
3. Wedging the catheter in the vessel being embolized
4. Gentle infusion of small quantities of embolic material
5. High resolution imaging devices for accurate monitoring of catheter position and flow of embolic materials
6. The use of radiopaque embolic material
7. Avoiding introduction of embolic material in stagnant systems (where spontaneous reflux is likely to occur)
8. Avoiding pressure injection of contrast media directly into embolized vessels
9. Avoiding embolization in patients with vasoconstriction, whether due to hypotension or vessel spasm

Choice of Materials and Methods for Specific Vascular Beds

Some general principles for the selection of materials can be stated. First, assuming equivalent risk, embolization should be avoided when an alternative method of treatment is avauable; while management of an infusion catheter requires more of the vascular radiologist's time, the complication rate of vasoconstrictor infusions is low [28]. Second, permanent occlusive materials should not be employed in situations in which shorter lasting materials are effective: thus. infusions is low [28]. Second, permanent occlusive materials should not be employed in situations in which shorter lasting materials are effective; thus, and safety of TVCO should be used [29]. Fourth, the time required to perform successful embolization may preclude its use in truly massive hemorrhage; while technically feasible, the risk to the patient associated with continuing massive blood loss and massive transfusion may far outweigh the risk of an operation and surgical ligation of the bleeding vessel. However, for certain causes of hemorrhage, (e.g., pelvic trauma or pelvic malignancy) transcatheter occlusive methods may be the only means of controlling bleeding [30].

he discussion that follows will outline our choices of materials for specific entities.

Tumors and Arteriovenous Malformations of the Head, Neck and Neuraxis

Complications of embolization of head and neck lesions relate almost entirely to reflux of emboli and ischemia of functioning cerebral tissue. The vascular supply to the face and pharynx is so rich that embolization to vessels other than those supplying the lesion is unlikely to be of significance. However, reflux from external carotid branches to the internal carotid artery can occur with potentially disastrous results. Embolization of internal carotid artery branches should be performed in high-flow systems so that embolic materials are directed away from normal tissue. Previously outlined methods to prevent reflux must be carefully applied. Berenstein and Kricheff [29] have carefully detailed the choice of materials for safe management of these lesions and recommend Gelfoam for use in presurgical devascularizations, reserving the permanent materials for arteriovenous malformations.

Gastrointestinal Hemorrhage

The issues regarding infusion vs. embolization in the treatment of gastrointestinal hemorrhage are well covered elsewhere in this issue. Gelfoam is the ideal material for TCVO control of gastrointestinal arteriocapillary hemorrhage because gastrointestinal hemorrhage is almost always a self-limited process. Small pieces of Gelfoam carefully introduced superselectively will produce excellent results and minimize the number of complications.

In three types of gastrointestinal hemorrhage problems, however, the use of materials other than Gelfoam may be indicated. The first is duodenal hemorrhage due to a large erosion of the gastroduodenal artery or pancreaticoduodenal arcades from ulcer disease. Gelfoam is usually inadequate in this situation, since it either passes through the vessel laceration or fails to occlude both sides of the circulation supplying the bleeding site. We have had excellent results with IBC introduced as close to the bleeding site as possible after being rendered radiopaque. The second and third indications for the use of materials other than Gelfoam are in the management of variceal hemorrhage via the transhepatic route. While the best results have been obtained by Widrich using Gelfoam soaked in sodium tetradecyl sulphate (Sotradecol) [3], IBC may be useful when difficulties are encountered in catheterizing the short gastric vessels from the splenic vein. Following embolization with Gelfoam in sodium tetradecyl sulfate, steel coils or detachable balloons may provide an additional measure of safety in the proximal occlusion of the major tributaries of the portal and splenic veins.

Intraabdominal Extraluminal Bleeding

Hemorrhage is a devastating complication in patients already critically ill. The use of absorbable materials is not recommended in post-pancreatic hemorrhage as the proleolytic emzymes released by massive lysis of pancreatic cells and autodigestion of surrounding tissues would also digest the Gelfoam causing recurrent hemorrhage. IBC, which has been life-saving in patients with this disastrous clinical circumstance, is the material of choice.

Hemorrhage Secondary to Trauma

TCVO is the primary mode of therapy for pelvic hemorrhage due to massive trauma [30]. It is also applicable in renal fracture, intrahepatic hemorrhage in the absence of free peritoneal rupture, laceration of muscular arteries resulting in expanding hematomas in the upper and lower extremities, and intrathoracic hemorrhage. Postoperative hemorrhage may

also be controlled. The use of Gelfoam is especially recommended in pelvic and extremity trauma and thoracic cavity bleeding. In order to preserve renal function, more precise control of renal bleeding points may be obtained with steel coils or detachable balloons. The choice of materials for hepatic trauma depends on the selectivity of catheterization that can be achieved, as discussed earlier. Where the site of hemorrhage can be reached with a large diameter catheter, Gelfoam is preferred; if coaxial systems are necessary, IBC or detachable miniballoons are suggested.

Hemorrhage from Tumors

Tumor hemorrhage, like some varieties of gastrointestinal hemorrhage, occurs in an abnormal tissue bed in which healing is not expected to occur. Therefore, the use of more permanent types of occlusion materials is indicated. Ivalon may be more suitable than Gelfoam as a particulate; IBC is often necessary when bleeding of larger magnitude is encountered. The choice of materials differs little for specific tumor types. In the presence of low grade (subangiographic) hemorrhage from the genitourinary tract presenting as either continued vaginal bleeding or hematuria in a patient with known pelvic or bladder malignancy, prophylactic occlusion of the hypogastric arteries may be of significant benefit [32]; Gelfoam or Ivalon is effective in these circumstances.

Preoperative or Palliative Occlusion of Tumor Blood Supply

Tumor palliation depends for its effect largely on acute dearterialization of the tumor with necrosis of the tumor bulk. It is necessary, therefore, to produce vessel occlusion within the tumor. Use of small particles, such as Gelfoam powder, Avitene, finely divided microspheres, or liquid polymers for capillary- or arterial-level occlusion is desirable. Ivalon is the most convenient particulate material to use, while the liquid materials are attractive in permitting a complete cast of the lesion to be formed, thus insuring more complete tumor ischemia. In order to allow reembolization if symptoms recur, the major vessels to the tumor should be left patent; since collateral blood flow will resupply the tumor if the major blood supply is interrupted, occlusion of the major vessels provides little advantage.

Preoperative reduction in vascularity requires both embolization at the precapillary level and proximal vessel occlusion. The precapillary occlusion decompresses the venous system by preventing collateral flow from reconstituting the circulatory pattern, and proximal vessel occlusion further reduces blood flow and provides additional safety during the resection, especially in bulky tumors where the surgeon may have difficulty isolating the feeding vasculature early in the resection. However, it is unwise to place embolic material too close to the origin of the renal artery since the material may be extruded into the aorta during cross-clamping of the vessel. Steel coils are ideal for the more proximal occlusion.

Hemoptysis

When hemoptysis is a complication of longstanding bronchiectasis, the bronchial arteries are hypertrophied and relatively simple to catheterize selectively enough to allow the safe introduction of embolic material [33]. Because of the profuse collateral supply in patients with bronchiectasis, precapillary level occlusion is necessary, either with small particles of Gelfoam or by use of a liquid polymer. In patients without longstanding inflammatory disease, safe catheterization may be impossible, but, should the coaxial technique allow safe peripheral placement of a small diameter catheter, liquid agents are suggested. In patients with bronchiectasis (from cystic fibrosis or longstanding chronic lung disease), maintaining patency of the proximal vessel, as in tumor embolization, may be desirable to allow repeat treatment of recurrent hemoptysis.

Arteriovenous Malformations of the Extremities

A staged approach to the treatment of large arteriovenous malformations is desirable. Since repeated embolizations may be necessary (unless the arteriovenous malformation is relatively small), proximal vessel occlusion should be avoided. Precapillary occlusion with particles of PVA or liquid polymer is necessary.

Pulmonary Arteriovenous Fistulas

Recent communications have advocated the use of both steel coils and detachable balloons for control of pulmonary arteriovenous fistulas [17, 34]. The latter seem ideal because of the precision with which they can be placed and because they remain tethered to the introducing catheter until detached. The major risk in dealing with pulmonary arteriovenous fistulas is systemic embolization of the occluding materials.

When the arteriovenous fistula cannot be selectively catheterized with the relatively large catheters necessary for introduction of the larger detachable miniballoon, steel coils may be successful since a smaller, more flexible catheter can be used with them. Occlusion of these lesions with liquids or particulate material should not be attempted because of the extreme danger of systemic embolization.

Arteriovenous Fistulae of the Abdominal Viscera

Posttraumatic, postoperative, and post-biopsy fistulae of the liver and kidney are easily managed with TCVO. Detachable balloons or steel coils are the materials of choice for these lesions, steel coils when the catheter can be easily placed at the mouth of the fistulae and detachable balloons when balloon flotation is necessary. There should be no need to resort to particulate materials, such as Gelfoam or PVA, except with very small fistulae. In such cases, a coaxial approach, using Gelfoam or a small amount of IBC, may be preferable. When the fistulae are large and occlusive control is thought to be dangerous because of possible embolization of materials to the venous circulation, temporary balloon occlusion of the feeding vessels may significantly reduce the risk of surgery. When the circulation to the organ in which the fistula is located can be safely interrupted for extended periods, inflation of the balloon in the angiographic suite is desirable, since this can precisely demonstrate the effects of the balloon catheter. For more critical applications, the precise volume necessary for balloon inflation can be determined in the angiographic suite and the balloon inflated in the operating room only if and when needed.

Visceral Artery Aneurysms

Intraparenchymal true and false aneurysms of the abdominal viscera must be ligated both proximally and distally to their origin. The ideal material for this is a liquid polymer, which can be introduced under very low pressure and allowed to flow through the lesion, with balloon control of inflow to prevent inadvertent distal embolization. As an alternative to liquid polymer in cases in which the catheter can be easily negotiated past the aneurysm, steel coils can be placed on either side of the aneurysm. If negotiation of the aneurysm is difficult, the use of flow-directed miniballoons may permit easy placement of an occluding device distal to the aneurysm.

Splenic Function Ablation

Strict attention to asepsis and antibiotic coverage are absolutely necessary to prevent abscess formation. The risk of sepsis is further reduced by partial embolization of the spleen in multiple sessions [35]. Capillary level occlusion with Ivalon is recommended, without proximal vessel occlusion. Where small catheters are necessary, IBC is second choice.

References

1. Grace, D.M., Pitt, D.F., Gold, R.E.: Vascular embolization and occlusion by angiographic techniques as an aid or alternative to operation. Surg. Gynecol. Obstet. 143:469–482, 1976
2. Miller, M.D., Johnsrude, I.S., Limberakis, A.J., Jackson, D.C., Pizzo, S., Thompson, W.M.: Clinical use of transcatheter electrocoagulation. Radiology 129:211–214, 1978
3. Doppman, J.L., Brown, E.M., Brennan, M.F., Spiegel, A., Marx, S.J., Auerbach, G.D.: Angiographic ablation of parathyroid adenomas. Radiology 130:577–582, 1979
4. Greenfield, A.J., Athanasoulis, C.A., Waltman, A.C., Le Moure, E.R.: Transcatheter embolization: Prevention of embolic reflux using balloon catheters. Am. J. Roentgenol. 131:651–655, 1978
5. Ring, E.J., Athanasoulis, C.A., Waltman, A.C., Margolies, M.N., Baum, S.: Arteriographic management of hemorrhage following pelvic fracture. Radiology 109:65–70, 1973
6. Wholey, M.H., Stockdale, R., Hung, T.K.: A percutaneous balloon catheter for the immediate control of hemorrhage. Radiology 95:65–71, 1970
7. Barth, K.H., Strandberg, J.D., White, R.I., Jr.: Long term follow-up transcatheter embolization with autologous clot, oxycel and gelfoam in domestic swine. Invest. Radiol. 12:273–280, 1977
8. White, R.I., Jr., Strandberg, J.V., Gross, G.S., Barth, K.H.: Therapeutic embolization with long-term occluding agents and their effects on embolized tissues. Radiology 125:677–687, 1977
9. Barth, K.H., Strandberg, J.D., Kaufman, S.L., White, R.I., Jr.: Chronic vascular reactions to steel coil occlusion devices. Am. J. Roentgenol. 131:455–458, 1978
10. Freeny, P.C., Mennemeyer, R., Kidd, R.C., Bush, W.H.: Long-term radiographic-pathologic follow-up of patients treated with visceral transcatheter occlusion using isobutyl 2-cyanoacrylate (Bucrylate). Radiology 132:51–60, 1979
11. Castaneda-Zuniga, W.R., Sanchez, R., Amplatz, K.: Experimental observations on short and long-term effects of arterial occlusion with Ivalon. Radiology 126:783–785, 1978
12. Diamond, N.G., Casarella, W.J., Bachman, D.M., Wolff, M.: Microfibrillar collagen hemostat: A new transcatheter embolization agent. Radiology 133:775–779, 1979
13. Luessenhop, A.J., Spence, W.T.: Artificial embolization of cerebral arteries. Report of use in a case of arteriovenous malformation. JAMA 172:1153–1155, 1960
14. Rösch, J., Dotter, C.T., Brown, M.J.: Selective arterial embolization. A new method for control of acute gastrointestinal bleeding. Radiology 102:303–306, 1972
15. Anderson, J.H., Wallace, S., Gianturco, C., Gerson, P.: "Mini" Gianturco stainless steel coils for transcatheter vascular occlusion. Radiology 132:301–303, 1979
16. Pevsner, P.H.: Micro-balloon catheter for superselective angiography and therapeutic occlusion. Am. J. Roentgenol. 128:225–230, 1977
17. White, R.I., Jr., Kaufman, S.L., Barth, K.H., DeCaprio, V., Strandbert, J.D.: Embolotherapy with detachable silicone balloons. Technique and clinical results. Radiology 131:619–627, 1979
18. Debrun, G, Legre, J., Kasbarian, M., Tapias, P.L., Caron, J.P.: Endovascular occlusion of vertebral fistulae by detachable balloons with conservation of the vertebral blood flow. Radiology 130:141–147, 1979
19. Gomes, A.S., Rysavy, J.A., Spadaccini, C., Probst, P., D'Souza, V., Amplatz, K.: The use of the bristle brush for transcatheter embolization. Radiology 129:345–350, 1978
20. Dotter, C.T., Goldman, M.L., Rösch, J.: Instant selective arterial occlusion with isobutyl 2-cyanoacrylate. Radiology 114:227–230, 1975
21. Freeny, P.C., Mennemeyer, R., Kidd, C.R., Bush, W.H.: Long-term radiographic-pathologic follow-up of patients treated with visceral transcatheter occlusion using isobutyl 2-cyanoacrylate (Bucrylate). Radiology 132:51–60, 1979
22. Doppman, J.L., Zapol, W., Pierce, J.: Transcatheter embolization with a silicone rubber preparation. Experimental observations. Invest. Radiol. 6:304–309, 1971
23. Doppman, J.L., Aven, W., Bowman, R.L., Wood, L.L., Girton, M.: A rapidly polymerizing polyurethane for transcatheter embolization. Cardiovasc. Radiol. 1:109–116, 1978
24. Trojanowski, J.Q, Harrist, T.J., Athanasoulis, C.A., Greenfield, A.J.: Hepatic and splenic infarctions: Complications and therapeutic transcatheter embolization. Am. J. Surg. 139:272–277, 1980
25. Rankin, R.N.: Gas formation after renal tumor embolization without abscess: A benign occurrence. Radiology 130:317–320, 1979
26. Spigos, D.G., Jonasson, O., Mozes, M., Capek, V.: Partial splenic embolization in the treatment of hypersplenism. Am. J. Roentgenol. 132:777–782, 1979
27. Bentson, J., Rand, R., Calcaterra, T., Lasjaunias, P.: Unexpected complications following therapeutic embolization. Neuroradiology 16:420–423, 1978
28. Greenfield, A.J., Waltman, A.C., Athanasoulis, C.A., Novelline, R.A., Dedrick, G.G.: Vasopressin in control of gastrointestinal hemorrhage: Complications of selective intra-arterial vs. systemic infusions (abstract). Gastroenterology 76, Part 2:1144, 1979
29. Berenstein, A., Kricheff, I.I.: Catheter and material selection for transarterial embolization: Technical considerations. Radiology 132:619–630, 1979
30. Athanasoulis, C.A., Harris, W.H., Stock, J.R., Waltman, A.C.: Arterial embolization to control pelvic hemorrhage. In: The Hip: Proceedings of the Seventh Open Scientific Meeting of the Hip Society, 1979. St. Louis, C.V. Mosby Co., 1980, pp. 247–259
31. Widrich, W.C., Johnson, W.C., Robbins, A.H., Nabseth, D.C.: Esophagogastric variceal hemorrhage. Arch. Surg. 113:1331–1338, 1978
32. Higgins, C.B., Bookstein, J.J., Davis, G.B., Galloway, D.C., Barr, J.W.: Therapeutic embolization for intractable chronic bleeding. Radiology 122:473–478, 1977
33. Fellows, K.E., Khaw, K.T., Schuster, S., Shwachman, H.: Bronchial artery embolization in cystic fibrosis: Technique and long term results. J. Pediatr. 95:959–963, 1979
34. Castaneda-Zuniga, W., Epstein, M., Zollikofer, C., Nath, P.H., Formanek, A., Ben-Shachar, G., Amplatz, K.: Embolization of multiple pulmonary artery fistulas. Radiology 134:309–310, 1980
35. Spigos, D.G., Jonasson, O., Mozes, M., Capek, U.: Partial splenic embolization in the treatment of hypersplenism. Am. J. Roentgenol. 132:777–782, 1979

Therapeutic Embolization with Detachable Balloons

Robert I. White, Jr., Klemens H. Barth, Stephen L. Kaufman, Vincent DeCaprio,*
and John D. Strandberg
The Russell H. Morgan Department of Radiology and Radiological Sciences and the Division of Comparative Medicine and the
Department of Pathology, The Johns Hopkins Medical Institutions, Baltimore, Maryland, USA

Abstract. In our first 18 months' clinical experience with embolization in the chest and abdomen using detachable balloons, successful results were obtained in 34 of 38 patients. One and 2-mm detachable silicone balloons, which can occlude vessels 4–8 mm in diameter, were employed. Prolonged balloon inflation was routinely achieved using iso-osmotic iodipamide meglumine as the filler and limiting inflation volumes to experimentally determined maximums. Improvements in introducer catheter design simplified delivery of the balloon into a variety of circulations.

Detachable balloons are not suitable for all embolization purposes, and they are frequently used in conjunction with other agents. When used properly, balloons produce a permanent occlusion that is extremely selective and potentially reversible up to a certain point in the procedure. The balloon technique enables the angiographer to occlude vessels at distances of 2–10 mm beyond the introducer catheter, thus avoiding the need for subselective catheterization and minimizing the dangers of inadvertent embolization.

Key words: Balloon occlusion technique – Embolism, therapeutic – Catheters and catheterization – Interventional radiology.

The successful results achieved with non-detachable balloon occlusion techniques in the neurovascular circulation provided the stimulus for the development of detachable and perfusion balloon technology [1–7]. Neuroradiologists and neurosurgeons initiated the use of balloon techniques because of the need for precise placement of embolic materials in the brain in order to prevent inadvertent embolization [8]. While non-detachable balloon catheters had also been used successfully to control hemorrhage in visceral arteries, cardiovascular radiologists began therapeutic embolization using a variety of particulate materials [9–12]. Embolization of the visceral circulation could be carried out with a greater margin of safety because of the availability of collateral arteries. Even in renal embolization, where selective occlusion was highly desirable because of a relative lack of collateral circulation, inadvertent embolization and infarction was associated with few permanent sequelae, except the loss of renal tissue. However, despite the relative safety of particulate material embolization in the visceral circulation, complications were reported [13–18].

In light of previous experimental and clinical studies we proposed the following criteria for safe and consistent therapeutic embolization [19–23]: (1) the embolization materials, because of their prolonged retention within the body, must be non-carcinogenic and non-toxic; (2) the occlusion produced must be extremely selective and reversible up to a certain point during the procedure, thus minimizing the risk of inadvertent embolization; and (3), since no embolic material is adequate alone in all instances, the therapeutic approach must allow the use of a combination of modalities. We realized that these criteria could not be uniformly achieved by embolization with particulate materials and that the detachable balloon techniques already used for neurovascular occlusion seemed to offer the best potential for an all-purpose occlusion technique for cardiovascular radiology.

Catheter and Technique

Serbinenko developed a silicone balloon for neurovascular occlusion in which long-term inflation was achieved by filling the balloon with a solidifying filler

* Biomedical Engineer, Becton-Dickinson Corporation, Rutherford, New Jersey 07070, USA

Supported in part by a grant from Becton-Dickinson Corporation, Rutherford, New Jersey 07070, USA
Address reprint requests to: R.I. White, Jr., M.D., Department of Radiology, Johns Hopkins Hospital, Baltimore, MD 21205, USA

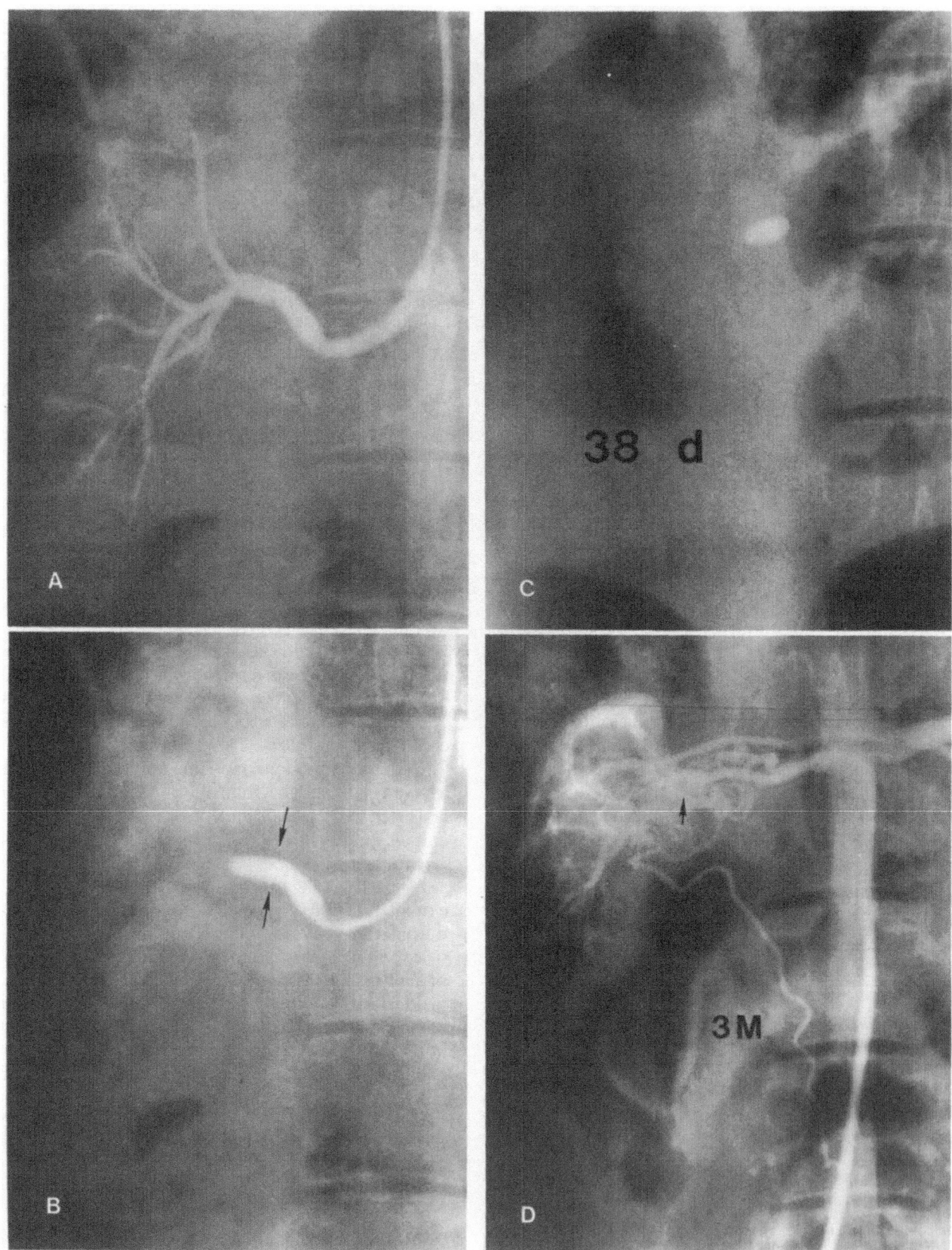

Fig. 1 A–D

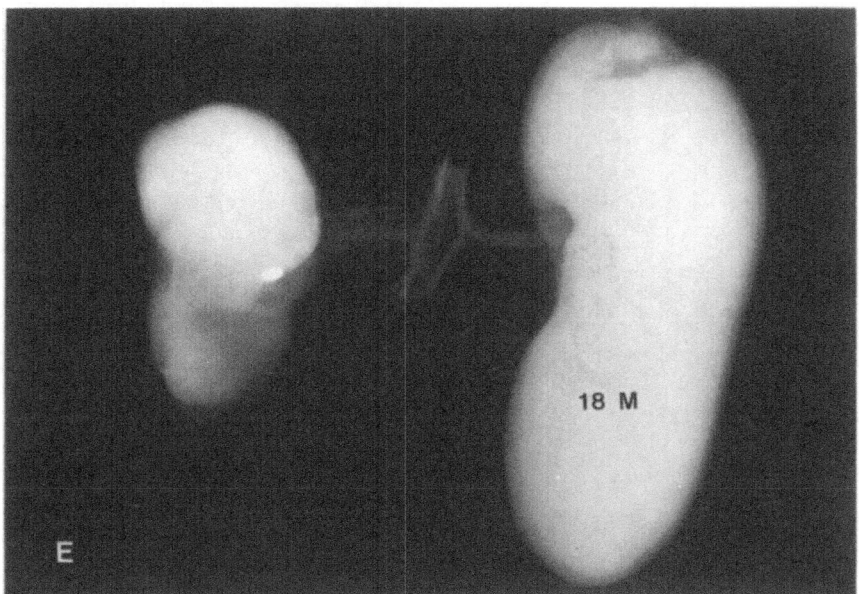

Fig. 1A–E. Experimental renal artery embolization with metrizamide-filled balloon in a pig followed for 18 months. **A** Control right renal arteriogram. **B** Immediate postembolization radiograph; arrows indicate the balloon, and the contrast material proximal to the balloon represents a small hand injection at the beginning of radiography. **C** After 38 days the balloon has assumed a more oval shape but remains unchanged in position and radiodensity. **D** Angiography at three months reveals marked atrophy of the right kidney. Extensive collaterals to the kidney arise proximal to the balloon (*arrow*), accounting for some preservation of renal function. **E** At the time of postmortem examination 18 months later, the balloon remains unchanged in position and radiodensity.

like liquid silicone [2]. Similarly, Debrun developed a latex balloon of improved design that appeared to seal when detached, but unfortunately contrast material leaked out of the balloon, leading to early deflation unless liquid silicone was used to fill the balloon [3, 8]. Additionally, preparation of the balloon by the angiographer was tedious, and latex was difficult to sterilize by conventional techniques. Clearly a balloon was needed that (1) could be consistently manufactured (preferably not by the angiographer the night before the procedure); (2) was self-sealing so that early deflation did not occur; and (3) required as filler only contrast material, which would serve as a radiopaque marker and allow for easy reversibility before detachment. Perfusion balloons, developed by neuroradiologists for superselective angiography and delivery of tissue adhesives in cerebrovascular arteriovenous malformations [2, 4, 6], were available, but it was realized that for cardiovascular applications a detachable balloon serving as an internal tourniquet was all that was required in the vast majority of instances. Biomedical engineers at Becton-Dickinson Corporation, stimulated by the experience of Serbinenko and the reports of Debrun, Kerber, and Pevsner, developed an improved and safer method of detaching balloons, using a self-sealing mechanism [2–4, 6].

Through two series of animal experiments and in vitro testing, the methods required to produce permanent balloon inflation and the length of time neces-

sary for the balloon to remain inflated to insure permanent vascular occlusion were determined [24–26]. Silicone proved to be semipermeable, and balloons filled with hyperosmotic contrast material underwent osmotic growth and early rupture. By using iso-osmotic contrast agents, permanent balloon inflation for up to 18 months was demonstrated in animals (Fig. 1). Results in animals embolized with balloons filled with contrast agents of varying osmolality demonstrated that if the balloons were inflated for 10 days or longer, 90% of the vessels remained permanently occluded, despite balloon deflation, as evidenced by follow-up angiography and postmortem examination three to six months later. Pathologic examination of the effects of silicone balloons on arterial walls demonstrated little evidence of inflammation. Furthermore, antegrade and retrograde thrombus formation occurred distally and proximally to the first branch point but not beyond. This assured permanent occlusion if the balloon deflated but did not lead to a long tail of thrombus with the possibility of proximal or distal embolization.

While the iso-osmotic metrizamide proved to be the radiopaque contrast material of choice as determined experimentally, its unavailability for intravascular studies in the United States led us to explore varying concentrations of the standard contrast material for intravenous cholangiography, iodipamide meglumine [30]. By diluting the latter contrast agent

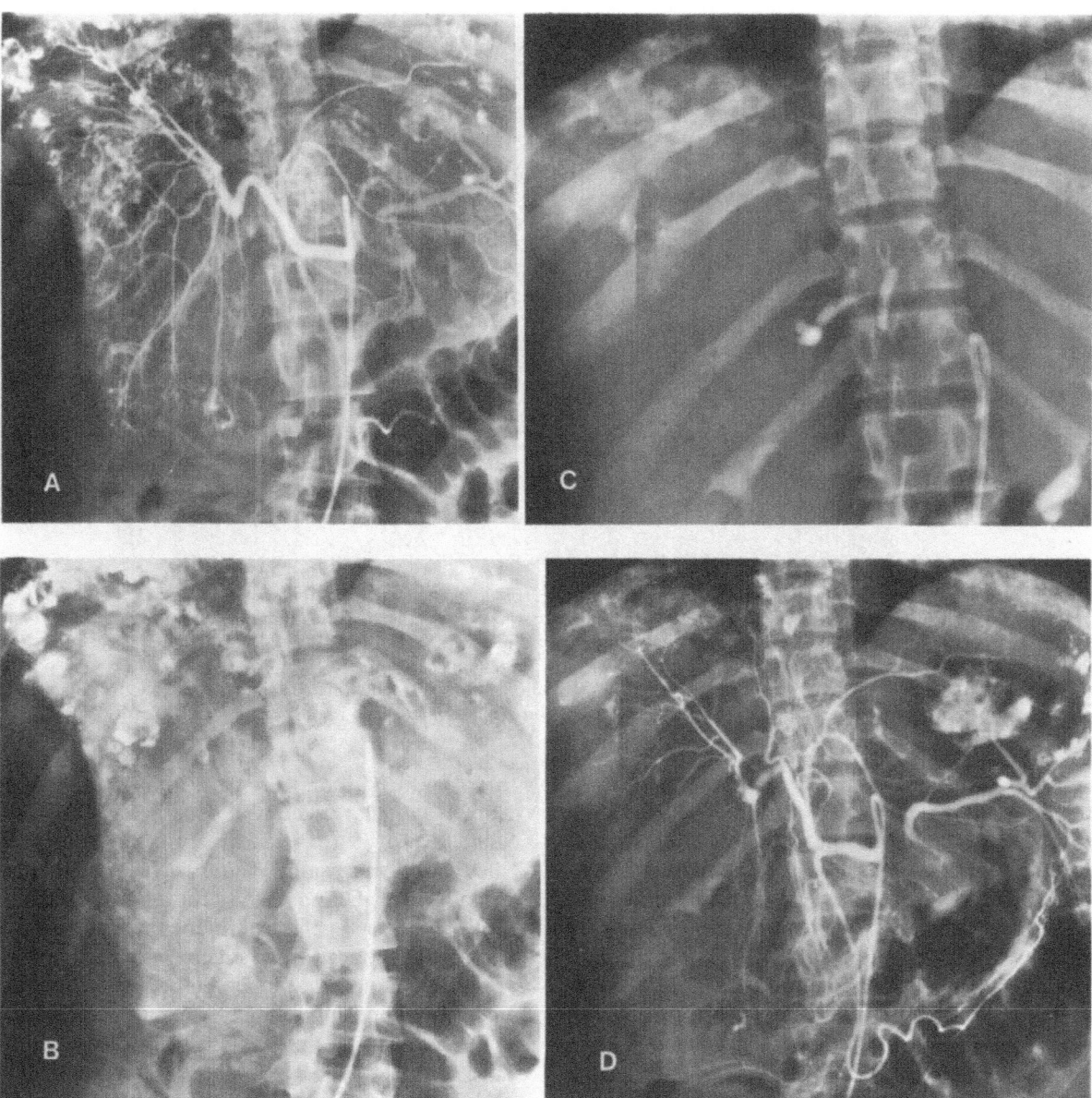

Fig. 2A–D. Patient with metastatic choriocarcinoma of the liver and acute subcapsular hematoma. **A** early and **B** late radiographs from the selective hepatic arteriogram reveal multiple hypervascular metastases and the typical concave deformity along the lateral border of the liver that is associated with subcapsular hematoma. **C** Three balloons were placed in branches of the right and left hepatic artery. **D** Folow-up angiogram reveals patency of the medial lobe branch of the left hepatic artery with collateral filling of the arteries to the lateral division of the left lobe. Residual patency of a portion of the right hepatic artery is also shown. A large splenic metastasis is seen in the left upper quadrant. The patient did well following balloon occlusion and was discharged after a course of chemotherapy.

by 50% with sterile water, a contrast material of suitable radiopacity and osmolality was achieved.

A number of modifications to the balloon-catheter delivery system were necessary before clinical studies were begun. A special coaxial catheter valve and coiling chamber were developed to ensure injection of the balloon catheter without knotting. The coaxial catheter valve allowed easy manipulation of the balloon catheter once it had been injected and permitted injection of saline and contrast material through the sidearm in order to keep the outer introducer catheter free of clot formation and to facilitate final positioning of the balloon. Introducer catheters of standard radiopaque polyethylene were satisfactory for many procedures and were often used in conjunction with a standard deflector wire. Nontapered, reinforced 6.5 French polyethylene catheters[1] with end-holes measuring 0.043 inches worked well for superselective visceral and external carotid catheterization.

It was determined that silicone balloons could be selectively placed coaxially through the introducer catheter and consistently detached. The balloons did not need to be detached until occlusion was confirmed by angiography through the introducer catheter. If the position of the balloon was unsatisfactory, it could be deflated before detachment and advanced more distally, withdrawn more proximally, or removed altogether. This provided us with a system that was reversible before release, and the flow direction of the balloon enabled us to achieve superselective positioning not often possible with other embolic materials. Radiopaque 2 French polyurethane tubing was adopted as the catheter material of choice, since it provided a small diameter catheter material of acceptable strength and flexibility.

Clinical Studies

After the animal experiments were completed in 1977, clinical embolization with the detachable silicone balloon was begun in January 1978 [27, 28]. The list of disorders that may be treated by these methods appears to grow with each passing month, but it is well to consider at this time our initial results during the first 18 months of balloon embolization ending July 1, 1979. During this 18-month period, 34 of 38 patients had arterial or venous occlusion performed successfully with the balloon, either alone or in conjunction with other agents. The first 16 patients have been previously reported [27, 28]. Clinical conditions requiring embolization were categorized in three major groups:

1. Hemorrhage, spontaneous, posttraumatic, and neoplastic.
2. Preoperative vascular embolization of large neoplasms to facilitate resection.
3. Congenital vascular malformations of the systemic, pulmonary, or venous circulations.

Hemorrhage

Hemorrhage occurring spontaneously, after trauma, or secondary to neoplastic erosion of arteries is easily controlled by transcatheter embolization (Fig. 2). Table 1 lists conditions in which detachable balloon embolization was successfully used to control bleed-

[1] Cook Incorporated, Bloomington, Indiana 47401, USA

Table 1. Cases in which hemorrhage was treated by balloon occlusion techniques (Jan. 1978–June 1979)

Disorder	No. of cases
Renal arteriovenous fistula	4
Pelvic fracture	2
False aneurysm[a] of the renal artery	1
False aneurysm of the vertebral artery	1
External carotid-jugular vein fistula	1
Bronchial artery (cystic fibrosis)	1
Duodenal ulcer	1
Post-hysterectomy	1
Carcinoma of the cervix	1
Liver (metastatic choriocarcinoma)	1
Total	14

[a] Unsuccessful balloon occlusion

ing. Posttraumatic bleeding in the pelvis, liver, and kidney is quite readily managed. While these conditions can also be effectively treated by embolization with particulate materials, balloons are much more selective, minimizing the danger of inadvertent embolization. In cases of posttraumatic fistulas, the detachable balloon technique is the method of choice, both because it is flow directed to the fistula and because particulate materials may pass through the fistula, resulting in embolization to the lung.

Our experience with hemoptysis is limited to one patient with cystic fibrosis, who has had permanent control of hemorrhage for the past 16 months [27]. Prior to the availability of transcatheter occlusion techniques, surgical ligation of the bronchial arteries had proved successful in controlling hemoptysis, and since detachable balloons represent an internal means of ligating arteries, it was reasoned that this technique would be as successful as the older surgical method. While consistent results have been achieved with Gelfoam embolization, there is always the possibility of inadvertent embolization into the aorta with this method [29]. Furthermore, embolization of particulate material in right-sided intercostal-bronchial trunks giving rise to spinal arteries is contraindicated, and while this variation only occurs in 5% of patients, careful angiographic studies are required to detect this anatomical feature. It is likely that detachable balloons can be used distal to the spinal artery takeoff without danger of occlusion of the spinal cord artery since retrograde thrombus only occurs back to the first branch point.

Cases in which there is gastrointestinal bleeding from larger arteries associated with duodenal and gastric ulcer and vasopressin-resistant diverticular bleeding have not been evaluated. This is due in part to the relative paucity of clinical material over the past 18 months and in part to the gastroduodenal artery frequently exceeding the maximum diameter of 4 mm, which is the limit of the current generation Mini-Balloon[2].

*Preoperative Vascular Embolization
of Large Neoplasms to Facilitate Resection*

In eight of nine patients, balloon occlusion has been successfully used to occlude the arterial supply to highly vascular neoplasms (Table 2). Preoperative arterial embolization of large renal cell carcinomas is routinely used to reduce operating time and blood loss. It is our impression that this form of therapy is helpful, and we have used detachable balloons along with a variety of other materials for this purpose. From two to four balloons are necessary to achieve satisfactory occlusion of large branch arteries supplying the tumor. For routine occlusion of large renal cell carcinomas, however, a combination of Gelfoam and coils can be employed as easily and with less expense.

For use before segmental liver resections, balloon occlusion techniques are ideal, since the balloons can be easily delivered into hepatic arterial branches to achieve a proximal occlusion. Our interest in studying balloons experimentally was generated because of the need for a safe material for the preoperative segmental occlusion of the hepatic circulation in a child with hepatoblastoma [30]. Figure 3 illustrates the use of segmental balloon occlusion for the resection of a large cavernous hemangioma of the liver.

For head and neck tumors, peripheral embolization of branches of the external carotid artery with material like microfibrillar collagen or Gelfoam, followed by proximal balloon occlusion to prevent reflux into the internal carotid artery and to reduce the amount of distal embolization required, are relatively simple and useful techniques [23]. Following distal embolization, the balloon can be placed immediately at the area of stasis, preventing any migration or redistribution of the embolic material to undesired sites.

Congenital Vascular Malformations

Goals for treatment of these uncommon but difficult management problems include either: (1) permanent

---

Table 2. Cases in which balloon occlusion techniques were employed for the preoperative devascularization of neoplasms (Jan. 1978–June 1979)[a]

Neoplasm	No. of cases
Hypernephroma	4
Cavernous hemangioma[b]	2
Ischial fibrous histiocytoma	1
Carotid body tumor	1
Meningioma	1
Total	9

[a] An unsuccessful attempt was also made to devascularize a small kidney with severe renal artery stenosis
[b] Unsuccessful attempt to detach balloon in 1 patient

Table 3. Cases in which balloon occlusion techniques were employed in the treatment of vascular malformations (Jan. 1978–June 1979)

Area of malformation	No. of cases
Pulmonary[a]	3
Pelvic	2
Scalp	2
Dural	1
Hemangioendothelioma	2
Testicular varicocele	4
Total	14

[a] The attempt to detach the balloon was unsuccessful in one large AVM

ablation, (2) transcatheter devascularization prior to surgical removal, or (3) palliation if resection is impossible. The choice of therapy is based primarily on the type of malformation and, secondarily, on its location. Congenital vascular malformations are conventionally divided into three types: systemic artery-to-systemic vein, pulmonary artery-to-pulmonary vein, and systemic vein (Table 3).

Systemic Artery-to-Systemic Vein. These malformations, which may occur intracerebrally, in the abdomen, or in the pelvis and extremities, are the most refractory to treatment. The arterial-venous connections are usually racimose and may be either large or much smaller and diffuse. Early (1960) attempts by Lussenhop at embolization of intracerebral arteriovenous malformations included blockage of feeding arteries by microspheres of varying sizes [31], while in another treatment approach, obliteration of the malformation rather than the feeding arteries was attempted [32, 33]. Ligation of arteries supplying the

---

[2] Becton-Dickinson Corporation, Rutherford, New Jersey 07070, USA

Fig. 3A–D. A and B Patient with large cavernous hemangioma of the right lobe of the liver. **C** A single balloon was placed in the right hepatic artery. **D** An angiogram immediately after the procedure demonstrates occlusion of the right hepatic artery. At the time of surgery, the hemangioma appeared decompressed and was resected with minimal blood loss.

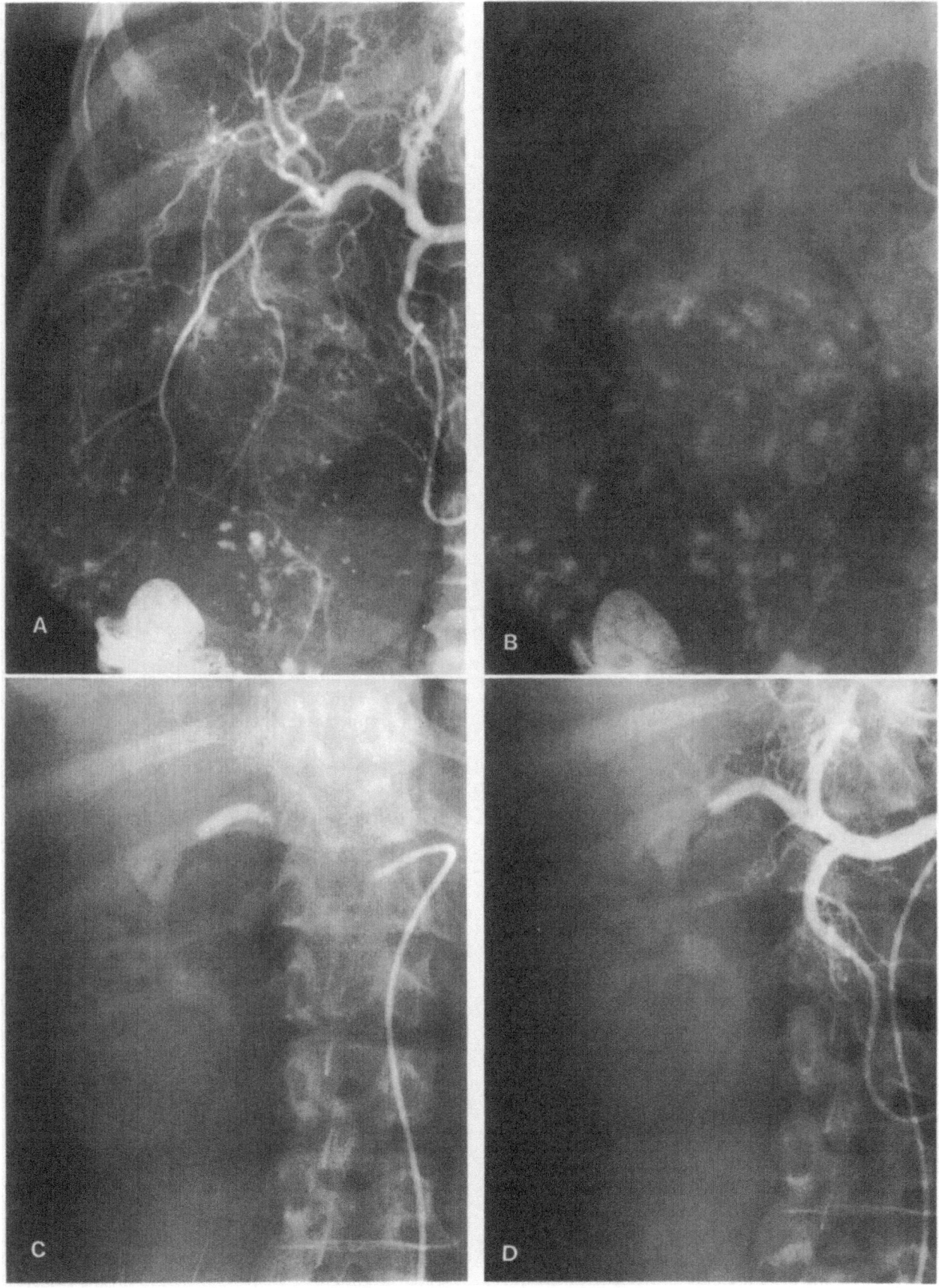

Fig. 3A–D

malformation, either surgically or with transcatheter embolization techniques, was associated with short-term palliation and the recurrence of the arteriovenous malformation coincident with the development of collateral arteries.

These malformations are best managed by transcatheter devascularization of major arteries followed by surgical removal. Unfortunately certain arteriovenous malformations are unresectable, because of their location, and in this group a variety of embolization techniques have been tried. In general, balloons offer no special advantage over other substances used for palliation except for their ease of delivery.

However, the successful preoperative balloon embolization of the feeding arteries to scalp arteriovenous malformations has shown that balloon techniques are extremely useful in reducing bleeding in this special group at the time of surgical removal (Fig. 4).

If balloons are used to block feeding arteries proximally without surgical resection or distal embolization, further attempts at palliation are precluded because the vessels are permanently blocked. Tissue adhesives and liquid silicone preparations hold promise in this difficult group of lesions, but as yet permanent ablation of congenital arteriovenous malformations has only rarely been accomplished by catheter techniques alone.

Pulmonary Artery-to-Pulmonary Vein. Pulmonary arteriovenous malformations (AVM) occur spontaneously or in association with Osler-Weber-Rendu Syndrome. They often develop in early adulthood and may progress both in size and number with age. Disability occurs through life-threatening hemoptysis, paradoxical embolization with cerebral infarction, or right-sided heart failure due to the hemodynamic burden of obligatory right-to-left shunting through the arteriovenous malformation. Traditionally, surgical resection has provided effective ablation of the largest of the malformations, but since the condition is progressive and often multiple areas of lung are involved, only limited resections are possible.

Transcatheter management of pulmonary AVMs has rarely been performed because all forms of particulate embolization are associated with the potential for passage of embolic material through the AVM and consequent systemic embolization. While wool coil embolization has been used successfully in this group of patients, particular care must be taken that the coil is large enough to occlude the AVM.

Detachable balloon techniques, because of their safety, are ideally suited for occluding pulmonary AVMs. The procedure is also facilitated by the flow-directed movement of the balloon once the introducer catheter has been positioned close to the feeding artery [34, 35]. Our limited experience has been gratifying, and we are convinced that when larger balloons are available, large pulmonary AVMs will be readily managed by these techniques. Our experience with several patients has indicated that, unlike systemic artery-to-vein fistulas, pulmonary AVMs once occluded remain so permanently without development of collateral arteries.

Systemic Vein – Varicocele. Testicular varicocele occurs in 3–10% of men and is associated with approximately 50% of all male infertility [36]. It is estimated that close to 12,000 surgical ligations for varicocele are performed annually in the United States. Transcatheter embolization with tissue adhesives or sclerosing agents and Gelfoam have produced long-term occlusion of varicoceles [37]. These techniques, however, require injection of unapproved substances and lack long-term follow-up.

Surgical ligation via an inguinal incision may be done on an outpatient basis, but unless venography is performed, collateral veins accounting for a recurrence rate of 10% may be overlooked. Retroperitoneal division and ligation of the testicular vein, which is a more definitive procedure, requires hospitalization and anesthesia. Transcatheter obliteration by detachable balloon techniques is permanent and easily performed on an outpatient basis. As the testicular vein in varicocele patients averages slightly greater than 6 mm in diameter, a special balloon capable of expanding to 8 mm in diameter was developed for use in these patients. Our experience in four patients to date has been most encouraging (Fig. 5). Follow-up radiographs and clinical examinations have confirmed persistent balloon inflation, and absence of the varicocele has been verified on serial examinations [38]. The balloons have not changed in position or size, and the only symptom has been mild scrotal tenderness lasting several days in two patients, presumably due to thrombosis of the varicocele. Pre-occlusion venograms have permitted precise placement of the balloon above any collateral veins that could cause recurrences. Results of semen analyses and clinical results regarding pregnancy are pending in these patients, and our long-term results and a detailed description of the technique are the subjects of another report [38].

Requirements for Successful Balloon Embolization and Analysis of Failures

Balloon embolization was unsuccessful in four of the first 38 patients, with three of the failures occurring

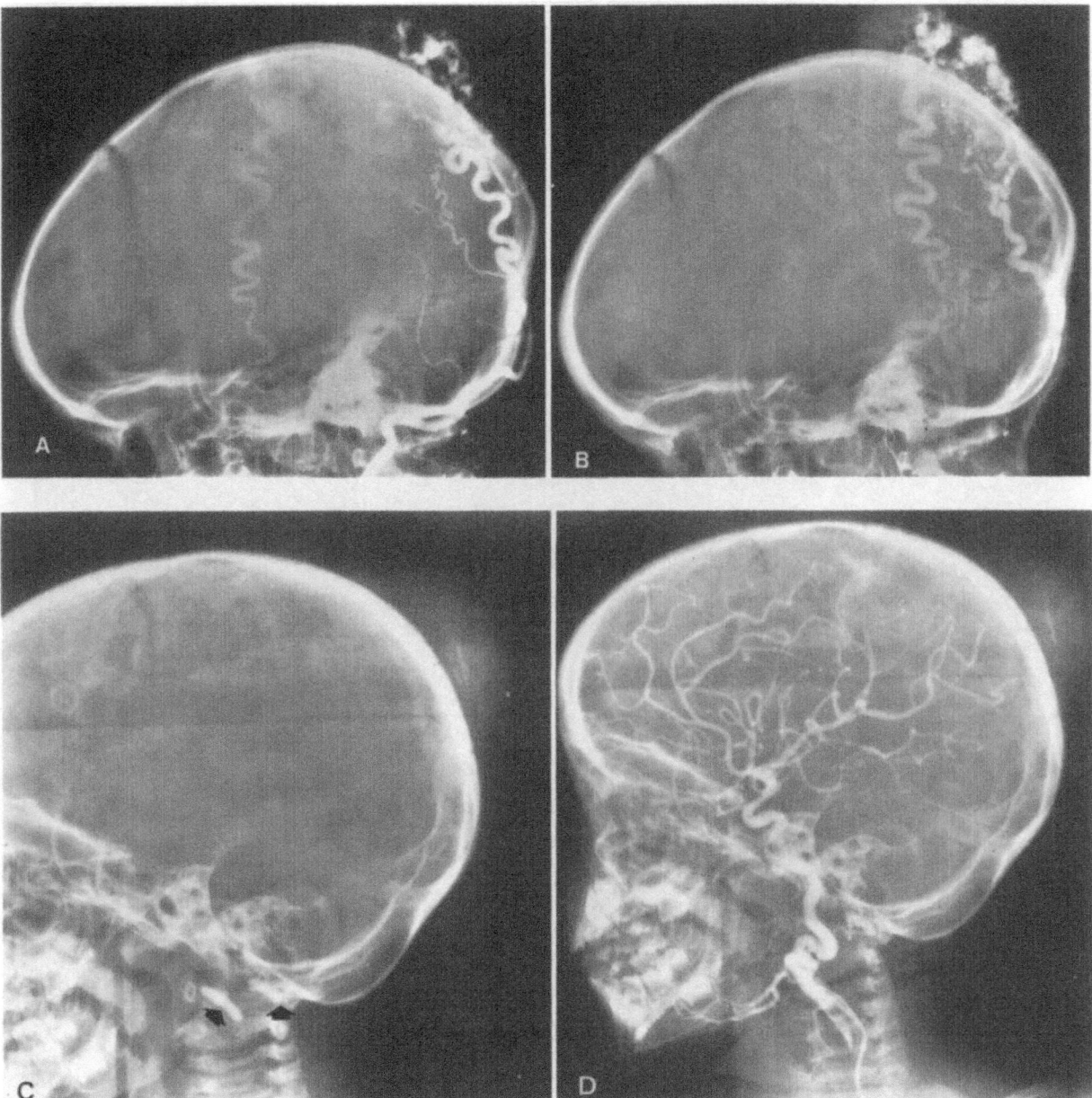

Fig. 4A–D. A and B Selective right occipital angiogram of a four-year-old patient with a large ulcerated scalp arteriovenous malformation (AVM). A diffuse blush and early venous filling are shown. **C** One balloon was placed in the occipital artery (*arrow*) and another was placed in the right external carotid artery immediately beyond the facial artery (arrow). **D** A right carotid arteriogram demonstrates no filling of the AVM. A balloon was also placed in the left occipital artery. The AVM was successfully resected with minimal blood loss.

during the first seven months we performed the procedure. Excessive tortuosity of the artery to be occluded and extreme length of the introducer catheter were responsible for an unsuccessful attempt to occlude branch hepatic arteries in a patient with a cavernous hemangioma of the right and left lobes of the liver. Because of tortuosity in the celiac axis, an axillary approach with a 5 French pediatric introducer catheter was required. The introducer catheter was quite easily advanced over a guidewire into the right and left branch hepatic arteries. The balloon catheter was injected and inflated easily, but multiple attempts to detach the balloon were unsuccessful. When the balloon catheter was pulled back it stretched, suggesting

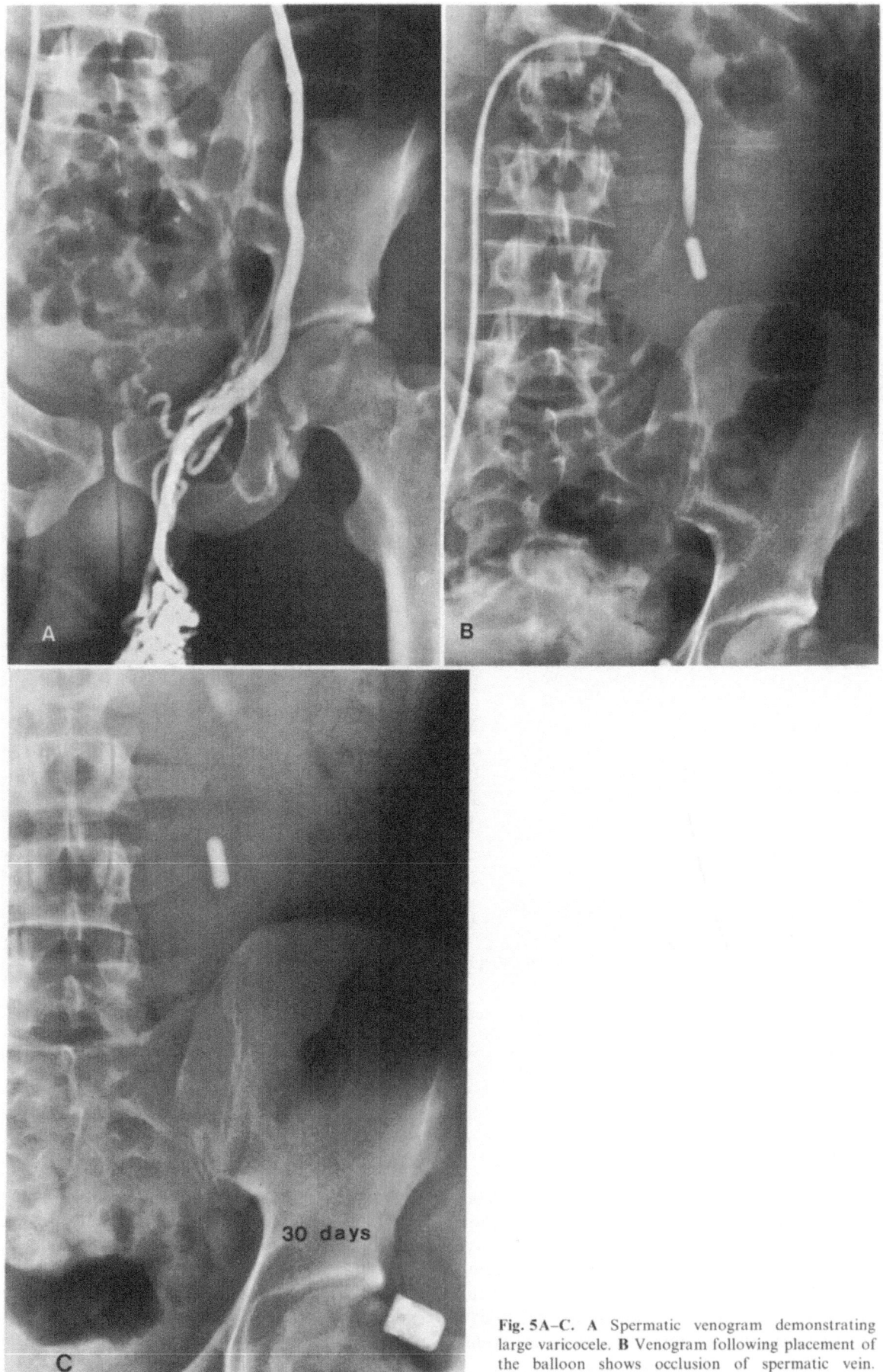

Fig. 5A–C. A Spermatic venogram demonstrating large varicocele. **B** Venogram following placement of the balloon shows occlusion of spermatic vein. **C** Thirty days later the balloon is unchanged in position, and the varicocele is no longer present.

that the detachment force was not transmitted distally to the balloon. Upon removal of the introducer catheter, it was noted that a severe kink had developed in the catheter at the point where it entered the celiac axis. A new introducer catheter was substituted, but the excessive tortuosity of the celiac and hepatic arteries still precluded successful detachment.

Excessive tortuosity of the artery or extreme length of the introducer catheter continue to be a cause of failures. We have learned to reduce any redundancy of the introducer catheter before detachment by pulling it back until the tip just begins to move from its selective position. This has led to successful balloon detachment in vessels with marked tortuosity. If the balloon does not detach easily as evidenced by continued stretching of the balloon catheter material, then the balloon should be deflated and the balloon catheter removed.

If the introducer catheter remains kinked, continued attempts to detach the balloon could lead to separation of the small balloon catheter within the introducer catheter. While we have not experienced this complication, it may occur, especially when the procedure is being learned. Should it occur, the introducer catheter could be pulled back into the aorta and the severed length of balloon catheter retrieved by standard catheter retrieval techniques. Familiarity with the forces normally required to detach balloons is best gained clinically during renal and pelvic artery or testicular vein embolizations, which we recommend as the starting point for learning the technique.

A second failure occurred because of our inability to cross a severe renal artery stenosis with the pediatric introducer catheter in a patient with a small kidney and renin-dependent hypertension. The development of special 6.5 French reinforced-wall catheters tapered to 5 French outer diameters at the tip has improved our ability to catheterize successfully all visceral arteries and the external carotid artery. These catheters have a nontapered endhole of 0.043 inches that readily allows passage of the 0.040 inch (1 mm) diameter Mini-balloon. Catheters with standard "Shepherd Crook," "Cobra," and "Head Hunter" shapes are now available.

Our third failure also occurred early in our experience when we were unable to place an introducer catheter in a lower pole segmental renal artery with a false aneurysm. The balloon was not flow directed into the branch because of lack of an associated fistula and we did not have torque-controlled catheters available to us at that time.

Our fourth failure occurred in a patient with a 1.0 cm left upper lobe pulmonary arteriovenous malformation. A prototype 2-mm-diameter (uninflated) balloon was inflated to its maximum diameter of 8 mm numerous times in the elongated upper lobe branch supplying the malformation. At no time could we achieve occlusion because of the size discrepancy, and the balloon was deflated and removed. This has occurred in other patients with pulmonary AVMs too large for both standard and prototype balloons. Careful assessment of vessel size on the diagnostic angiogram will help avoid unsuccessful attempts to occlude arteries too large for the balloons. Of course, the ability to test occlude a pulmonary AVM before balloon detachment is an important safety feature not provided by other embolic materials.

If the vessel to be occluded is not of nearly uniform diameter in the segment where the balloon is placed, firm placement and occlusion will not be achieved. For example, with patent ductus arteriosus, the conical narrowing throughout the length of the ductus may not allow safe occlusion with a cylindrically shaped balloon of uniform diameter, since the inflated balloon can easily back up into the aorta or pass into the pulmonary artery. The feasibility of long-term occlusion of systemic artery-to-pulmonary artery connections has been demonstrated with surgically created subclavian-pulmonary artery shunts [39]. The characteristically uneven diameter of patent ductus arteriosus is also shared by some bronchial arteries in patients with pulmonary valve atresia, ventricular septal defect, and direct bronchial artery-to-pulmonary artery connections [40].

Looking Toward the Future

Soon after clinical embolization was begun it was realized that the maximum vessel diameter that could be occluded was 4 mm. This led to the development of a 2 mm diameter balloon that could be expanded to greater than 8 mm. While this offered a system for occluding the larger arteries and even some veins, its use required introducer catheters larger than 8 French, making the employment of a percutaneous approach less attractive in some patients. In order to keep the introducer catheter size to a minimum (5 French, ideally), a balloon material permitting greater expansion would have to be developed and proven safe for long-term implantation.

A second area of concern is that of vessel tortuosity. Difficulties in navigation and detachment along tortuous routes presents complex problems involving the characteristics of blood flow and the physical properties of catheter material. Ideally, we would like the most flexible catheter material available without compromising strength, thus allowing the catheter to offer the least resistance to blood flow while maintaining enough strength and stiffness to hold up under detachment. Additionally, because the balloon catheter must be detached coaxially, through the introducing catheter, the sliding frictional properties of the materials are extremely important. Vessel tortuosity tends to amplify the force required to effect detachment. Although only a few grams of force are normally required to detach an inflated balloon from its catheter, several times that force may be required to detach the balloon along a highly tortuous route where the balloon catheter presses against the introducer catheter at several bends. If tortuosity is excessive, enough force may be generated to break the catheter during detachment. If the balloon catheter material is made too flexible, so that it becomes "rubbery," excessive stretching will occur during detachment and essentially no force will be transmitted to the balloon.

It is most probable that all the problems associated with balloon embolization cannot be solved with one "universal" balloon catheter system. Because of the great assortment of indications for therapeutic embolization, the "state of the art" balloon system will eventually comprise balloons of various shapes and elongations, having either stiff or flexible catheters attached. Additionally, an array of introducer catheters will be developed, no longer designed simply for the introduction or withdrawal of fluids, but also designed to allow passage of one of several types of balloon catheters selectively and with maximum safety. The current system must be viewed as a technique in evolution. Although we now consider it the safest and most controllable catheter technique for occluding vessels, our experience has pointed the way to future development.

Acknowledgements. We gratefully acknowledge the secretarial assistance of Mrs. Olga Carr in preparation of this manuscript.

References

1. Prolo, D.K., Handbery, J.W.: Intraluminal occlusion of a carotid-cavernous fistula with a balloon catheter. J. Neurosurg. 35:237–242, 1971
2. Serbinenko, F.A.: Balloon catheterization and occlusion of major cerebral vessels. J. Neurosurg. 41:125–145, 1974
3. Debrun, G., Lacour, P., Caron, J.P., Hurth, M., Comoy, J., Keravel, Y., Laborit, G.: Experimental approach to the treatment of carotid cavernous fistulas with an inflatable and isolated balloon. Neuroradiology 9:9–12, 1975
4. Kerber, C.: Balloon catheter with a calibrated leak. Radiology 120:547–550, 1976
5. DiTullio, M.V. Jr., Rand, R.W., Frisch, E.: Development of a detachable vascular balloon catheter: A preliminary report. Bull. Los Angeles Neurol. Soc. 41:2–5, 1977
6. Pevsner, P.H.: Micro-balloon catheter for superselective angiography and therapeutic occlusion. Am. J. Roentgenol. 128:225–230, 1977
7. Guillaume, J., Roulieau, J.: Experimental embolization with inflatable and releasable balloons in dogs. Neuroradiology 14:85–88, 1977
8. Debrun, G., Lacour, P., Caron, J.P., Hurth, M., Comoy, J., Keravel, Y.: Detachable balloon and calibrated-leak balloon techniques in the treatment of cerebral vascular lesions. J. Neurosurg. 49:635–649, 1978
9. Wholey, M.H., Stockdale, R., Hung, T.K.: A percutaneous balloon catheter for immediate control of hemorrhage. Radiology 95:65–71, 1970
10. Rösch, J., Dotter, C.T., Brown, M.J.: Selective arterial embolization: A new method for control of acute gastrointestinal bleeding. Radiology 102:303–306, 1972
11. Margolies, M.N., Ring, E.J., Waltman, A.C., Kerr, W.S., Jr., Baum, S.: Arteriography in the management of hemorrhage from pelvic fractures. N. Engl. J. Med. 287:317–321, 1972
12. Almgård, L.E., Fernström, I., Haverling, M., Ljungquist, A.: Treatment of renal adenocarcinoma by embolic occlusion of the renal circulation. Br. J. Urol. 45:474–479, 1973
13. Woodside, J., Schwarz, H., Bergreen, P.: Peripheral embolization complicating bilateral renal infarction with Gelfoam. Am. J. Roentgenol. 126:1033–1034, 1976
14. Gang, D.L., Dole, N.K., Adelman, L.S.: Spinal cord infarction following therapeutic renal artery embolization. JAMA 237:2841–2842, 1977
15. Tegtmeyer, C.J., Smith, T.H., Shaw, A., Barwick, K.W., Kattwinkel, J.: Renal infarction: A complication of Gelfoam embolization of a hemangioendothelioma of the liver. Am. J. Roentgenol. 128:305–307, 1977
16. Braf, Z.F., Koontz, W.W., Jr.: Gangrene of bladder: Complication of hypogastric artery embolization. Urology 9:670–671, 1977
17. Hietala, S.: Urinary bladder necrosis following selective embolization of the internal iliac artery. Acta Radiol. [Diagn.] (Stockh.) 19:316–320, 1978
18. Chuang, V.P.: Nonoperative retrieval of Gianturco coils from abdominal aorta. Am. J. Roentgenol. 123:996–997, 1979
19. Osterman, F.A., Jr., Bell, W.R., Montali, R.J., Novak, G.R., White, R.I., Jr.: Natural history of autologous blood clot embolization in swine. Invest. Radiol. 11:267–276, 1976
20. Barth, K.H., Strandberg, J.D., White, R.I., Jr.: Long term follow-up of transcatheter embolization with autologous clot, Oxycel and Gelfoam in domestic swine. Invest. Radiol. 12:273–279, 1977
21. White, R.I., Jr., Strandberg, J.V., Gross, G.S., Barth, K.H.: Therapeutic embolization with long-term occluding agents and their effects on embolized tissues. Radiology 125:677–687, 1977
22. Barth, K.H., Strandberg, J.D., Kaufman, S.L., White, R.I., Jr.: Chronic vascular reactions to steel coil occlusion devices. Am. J. Roentgenol. 131:455–458, 1978
23. Kaufman, S.L., Strandberg, J.D., Barth, K.H., White, R.I., Jr.: Transcatheter embolization with microfibrillar collagen in swine. Invest. Radiol. 13:200–204, 1978
24. White, R.I., Jr., Ursic, T.A., Kaufman, S.L., Barth, K.H., Kim, W., Gross, G.S.: Therapeutic embolization with detachable balloons: Physical factors influencing permanent occlusion. Radiology 126:521–523, 1978
25. Kaufman, S.L., Strandberg, J.D., Barth, K.H., Gross, G.S., White, R.I., Jr.: Therapeutic embolization with detachable silastic balloon: Long term effects in swine. Invest. Radiol. 14:156–161, 1979
26. Barth, K.H., White, R.I., Jr., Kaufman, S.L., Strandberg, J.D.: Metrizamide, the ideal radiopaque filler for detachable silastic balloon embolization. Invest. Radiol. 14:35–40, 1979
27. White, R.I., Jr., Kaufman, S.L., Barth, K.H., DeCaprio, V.,

Strandberg, J.D.: Therapeutic embolization with detachable silicone balloons: Early clinical experience. JAMA 241:1257–1260, 1979

28. White, R.I., Jr., Kaufman, S.L., Barth, K.H., DeCaprio, V., Strandberg, J.D.: Embolotherapy with detachable silicone balloons: Technique and clinical results. Radiology 131:619–627, 1979

29. Remy, J., Arnaud, A., Fardou, H., Giraud, R., Voisin, C.: Treatment of hemoptysis by embolization of bronchial arteries. Radiology 122:33–37, 1977

30. Shermeta, D.W., Golladay, E.S., White, R.I., Jr.: Preoperative occlusion of the hepatic artery with isobutyl 2-cyanoacrylate for resection of the "unresectable" hepatic tumor. Surgery 83:319–322, 1978

31. Luessenhop, A.J., Spence, W.T.: Artificial embolization of cerebral arteries: Report of use in a case of arteriovenous malformation. JAMA 172:1153–1155, 1960

32. Sano, K., Jimbo, M., Saito, I., Terao, H., Hirakawa, K.: Artificial embolization with liquid plastic. Neurol. Medicochir. 8:198, 1966

33. Doppman, J.L., Zapol, W., Pierce, J.: Transcatheter embolization with a silicone rubber preparation: Experimental observations. Invest. Radiol. 6:304–309, 1971

34. White, R.I., Jr., Barth, K.H., Kaufman, S.L., Terry, P.B.: Detachable silicone balloons: Results of experimental study and clinical investigations in hereditary hemorrhagic telangiectasia. Ann. Radiol. (Paris) 23:338–340, 1980

35. Terry, P.B., Barth, K.H., Kaufman, S.L., White, R.I., Jr.: Balloon embolization for treatment of pulmonary arteriovenous fistulas. N. Engl. J. Med. 302:1189–1190, 1980

36. Walsh, P.C.: A new cause of male infertility (editorial). N. Engl. J. Med. 300:253–254, 1979

37. Zeitler, E.: Selective sclerotherapy of the internal spermatic vein in patients with varicoceles. Cardiovasc. Intervent. Radiol. 3:166–169, 1980

38. Walsh, P.C., Barth, K.H., Kaufman, S.L., White, R.I., Jr.: Technic and long term results of percutaenous occlusion of varicocele with detachable silicone balloons. Presented at the American Urological Association Meeting, San Francisco, Calif., May 22, 1980

39. White, R.I., Jr., Magee, P.G., Roland, J.-M., Strandberg, J.D., Donahoo, S.: Closure of systemic-pulmonary shunts by detachable silastic balloon embolization (abstract). Circulation 58 (Suppl. 2): II-71, 1978

40. McGoon, M.D., Fulton, R.E., Davis, G.D., Ritter, D.G., Neill, C.A., White, R.I., Jr.: Systemic collateral and pulmonary artery stenosis in patients with congenital pulmonary valve atresia and ventricular septal defect. Circulation 56:473–479, 1977

Comment

Materials and Methods for Transcatheter Vascular Occlusion: Some Personal, Practical Views

Josef Rösch, Frederick S. Keller, and Charles T. Dotter

Department of Diagnostic Radiology, School of Medicine, University of Oregon Health Sciences Center, Portland, Oregon, USA

In his paper, Greenfield reviews in detail the materials, devices, methods, and appropriate uses of transcatheter therapeutic vascular occlusion. In another report, White and coworkers focus on a specific and promising approach to selective vascular occlusion, the detachable balloon. Over 150 publications in the 1979 scientific literature emphasize the importance and diversity of methods now available for transcatheter vascular occlusion. The following comments reflect our personal views, based on a decade of experience in this field.

Many means are available for percutaneous transcatheter vascular occlusion. Occlusive materials of endogenous or exogenous origin range from liquids to various solid particles with differing degrees of absorbability. Occlusive or obstructive devices include simple balloon catheters, metallic coils or brushes, detachable balloons, intracaval filters, and closure devices tailored for specific congenital lesions.

Technical choices are influenced by many important factors. Among these are: (1) the type of lesion to be occluded, its location, size and configuration, as well as the character of its vessels, including primary and collateral arterial feeders and draining veins; (2) the desired duration of occlusion; (3) catheter accessibility; (4) the benefits and the risks of intended (or unintended) occlusion; (5) availability of suitable occlusive materials or devices; (6) the angiographer's familiarity with their use; and (7) cost which, unfortunately, must also be considered.

Ideally, all vasoocclusive agents, whether used for short, prolonged, or permanent occlusion, should be nontoxic and noncarcinogenic. They should be reasonably easy to use without endangering uninvolved

tissues and organs; radiopaque, so that their application can be controlled; and readily available in suitable, sterile form. A single, universal, occlusive means, appropriate under all circumstances for all lesions, neither exists nor can be developed. Therapeutic angiographers must, therefore, be familiar with a variety of means, and able to choose and use them as indicated by case-specific needs and circumstances. Fortunately, it is not necessary to have experience with all, since several are capable of equivalent results. A suitably chosen few will suffice; increasing familiarity with their use will, through experience, improve effectiveness and safety.

There are, and always will be, differing opinions and technical preferences within the ranks of therapeutic angiographers, since there are many means to the common goal: safe and effective therapeutic transcatheter vascular occlusion.

After exploring a host of occluding materials, devices, and techniques and their combinations, we have come to rely upon a few, mostly conventional, approaches.

Balloon catheters of various sizes offer us effective, safe means for temporary, immediately reversible, nonoperative control over massive bleeding, even from the largest of arteries.

For medium term (days to weeks) occlusion, as in the control of nontumorous bleeding from smaller arteries, arterioles, and capillaries, we rely heavily on Gelfoam. In powder form, it is used for selective left gastric embolization to treat mucosal or small vessel hemorrhage and traumatic pelvic bleeding from small vessels. Mixed into a slurry with contrast medium, its fluoroscopically monitored delivery can be controlled with little risk of misdirection or reflux into non-target areas. We have not encountered ischemic, embolic, or other significant complications in 36 patients treated this way. For bleeding from medium-sized vessels, pieces of malleable Gelfoam

Address reprint requests to: J. Rösch, M.D., Department of Diagnostic Radiology, School of Medicine, University of Oregon Health Sciences Center, Portland, OR 97201, USA

suspended in contrast agent are injected by catheter directly into the bleeding vessels or their feeders. Although we have not used autologous clot embolization for seven years, it can be considered as a last resort when the desired catheter position cannot be achieved and the need for controlling serious hemorrhage outweighs the risk of imprecisely controlled embolization.

Permanent mahular occlusion is most often used in the palliative management of tumors, particularly malignancies. Associated problems, such as bleeding, hematuria, pain, and undesired endocrinologic function, often respond to occlusion either by a combination of Gelfoam and Gianturco coilspring occluders or by cyanoacrylate tissue adhesive. Readily available, easily used combinations of Gelfoam and coilsprings are usually sufficient. In hypervascular tumors, especially those with arteriovenous shunts, we prefer to use Gelfoam pieces rather than powder. Following Gelfoam embolization, the coilspring occlusion of *all* tumor-feeding vessels allows complete, permanent devascularization. For most indications, the availability, easily used combinations of Gelfoam and coilsprings are usually sufficient. In hypervascular tumors, especially those with arteriovenous shunts, we prefer to use Gelfoam pieces rather than powder. Following are literally hundreds of times more costly.

Special considerations bear upon the transcatheter treatment of angiomas, especially arteriovenous malformations. Detachable balloons offer the best approach for treating large, direct, arteriovenous fistulas in, for example, the pulmonary circulation. Here, predetachment testing and balloon retrievability insure selective occlusion with minimal loss of functioning lung and offer significant technical advantages.

In complex, systemic arteriovenous malformations, as opposed to direct fistulas, the anatomic situation and its management are different. The occlusion of all grossly apparent feeding arteries is of limited value in most systemic arteriovenous malformations with multiple feeders and an extensive central vascular nidus. These complex lesions offer a real challenge to the therapeutic angiographer, since unless their entire vascular nidus is occluded, they soon acquire new feeders and recur, often larger in size. After a long, usually disappointing experience with various other means of occlusion, we have found isobutyl 2-cyanoacrylate mixed with iophendylate (Pantopaque) best suited for such lesions. In view of the currently restricted availability of cyanoacrylate and the need for practical experience in its use, the occlusive therapy of diffuse, systemic arteriovenous malformations is, regrettably but necessarily, limited to certain institutions.

In the use of any technique for therapeutic transcatheter occlusion, we place a continuing emphasis on the avoidance of complications. Proximally occluding catheters are of value in preventing inadvertently misdirected emboli. Their combination with venous balloon catheters to occlude draining veins can prevent pulmonary embolization.

The foregoing technical considerations, while both relevant and current, are far from the last words on the subject. Bureaucracy and inflation not withstanding, technical improvements will surely continue to evolve. The timeless, yet moving, "bottom line" will continue to be defined and redefined by the inventiveness, procedural skill, and clinical judgment of many angiographers and their important allies in the catheter industry.

Editor's Note

When Gelfoam is used in powder form–as suggested by Rösch, Keller, and Dotter–great caution should be exercised to avoid tissue infarction. Gelfoam pledgets lodge proximally, while powder occludes small arterioles and capillaries and may result in tissue necrosis.

Vessel Occlusion with Transcatheter Electrocoagulation

William M. Thompson[1] and Irwin S. Johnsrude[2]

Departments of Radiology, Duke University Medical Center,[1] Durham, North Carolina, and Pitt County Memorial Hospital,[2] Greenville, North Carolina, USA

Abstract. Transcatheter intravascular electrocoagulation for therapeutic occlusion of vessels has been experimentally developed and successfully used clinically as an alternative to, and in conjunction with, more routine methods of vessel occlusion. A constant current power source and a steelguide wire anode are used for the occlusion. The subject is grounded with a standard bovie plate insulated from the skin by a highly lubricated sponge. Permanent occlusion of strategic vessels at accurately controlled sites has been achieved with little risk of embolization of nontarget areas. There has been minimal damage to vessel walls, and complete occlusion has been possible despite heparinization and/or thrombocytopenia. One limitation is the inconstant ability to position the anode precisely at the desired site of occlusion. Also, a long time may be required (up to one hour) to occlude larger vessels with presently available anodes. Wider use must await refinements in development of the anode material and in its delivery system.

Key words: Arteries, therapeutic blockade – Catheters and catheterization – Electrocoagulation – Interventional radiology.

Address reprint requests to: W.M. Thompson, M.D., Department of Radiology, Duke University Medical Center, Durham, NC 27710, USA

Therapeutic transcatheter occlusion of vessels is a well-accepted technique for controlling hemorrhage, infarcting vascular tumors, and reducing the blood supply to arteriovenous malformations. Many methods have been developed, ranging from infusion of drugs to injection of a variety of materials [1, 2, 4–6, 9–13, 17, 21–23, 29, 30, 34–37]. While the effectiveness of these procedures for vessel occlusion is well established, all have significant risks, most importantly, the accidental occlusion of a nontarget vessel.

In 1953, Sawyer and Pate [28] showed that small amounts of direct current applied across a vessel wall produced thrombosis and concluded that the current interfered with the normal bioelectric phenomena of the vessel wall. Phillips applied this principle to occlude the upper intestinal arteries of dogs [24] and subsequently showed that transcatheter electrocoagulation (TCEC) could be used to occlude surgically created arteriovenous fistulae [25].

Several other mechanisms have been proposed to explain why thrombosis occurs when direct current is applied across a vessel wall via a luminal anode. Possible physiological mechanisms are: (1) platelet attraction to the positive electrode, (2) intimal damage, and (3) release of clotting factors [28, 33]. The electrochemical mechanisms proposed are: (1) change in pH, (2) thermal damage, (3) precipitation of protein and

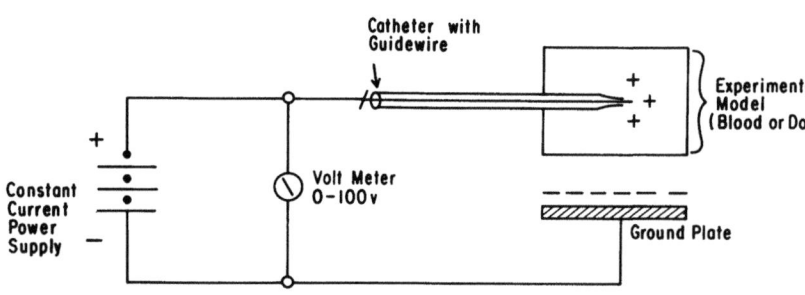

Fig. 1. Circuit diagram for dc coagulation. The battery represents the constant current power source. The catheter and electrode are drawn in the blood or dog's artery. (Reprinted with permission from [12].)

inorganic salts, and (4) diffusion of toxic reaction end-products or intermediates into the tissues [7, 8]. The exact role, if any, of each of these mechanisms is unknown, but a combination of effects probably occurs.

Methods (Fig. 1)

Based on our laboratory and clinical work, we have developed the following TCEC technique. A constant current power supply[1] is used to deliver 15 ma of direct current (dc) for 15 to 30 minutes. The positive electrode is a standard stainless steel guidewire insulated from the vessel by a standard angiographic catheter without sideholes. The catheter is introduced through a femoral sheath that permits multiple catheter exchanges. The tip of the anode protrudes from the catheter by 3–5 mm and touches the vessel wall. The cathode is a standard bovie plate separated from the subject by a highly conductive sponge.[2] Voltage across the subject is constantly monitored using a volt meter.[3] If the voltage limit of the constant current dc power supply (110 volts) is exceeded, this indicates a marked increase in resistance. Since this usually means a break in the circuit, the procedure is stopped and all connections are checked. Occasionally, however, the anode may have slipped back into the catheter, or if TCEC has been performed for more than 25 minutes, the tip of the anode may have broken due to electrolysis. The catheter insulating the anode is not flushed during the procedure. For post-occlusion angiograms, the catheter is replaced through the femoral sheath. In clinical situations, patients who are not bleeding are anticoagulated with heparin (45 units/per kilogram).

Experimental Work

In 1977, in vitro and in vivo experiments showed that the clot size and extent of thrombosis of vessels in which TCEC was applied were directly related to the total amount of current [31] (Fig. 2). Surgically created splenic hemorrhages were controlled in eight of nine dogs, with the vessels remaining occluded for up to 15 weeks after TCEC. At autopsy the vessels showed a small amount of initimal damage at the occlusion site (Fig. 3). These experiments suggested that thrombosis may be the result of both intimal damage and platelet attraction to the positive electrode.

The following year, we showed that TCEC produced substantial clots in thrombocytopenic canine blood in vitro [32]. Also, the splenic artery remained occluded for up to four weeks in three dogs following restocetin-induced thrombocytopenia. The results suggest that TCEC might be effective for occluding vessels in patients with platelet-poor blood. Subsequent studies indicated that thrombosis also occurs in heparinized blood [32].

A disadvantage of the stainless steel anode is that it undergoes electrolysis and occasionally breaks off in the thrombus [7, 15, 31–33] (Fig. 4). In vitro testing suggested that an intraarterial bipolar platinum electrode might achieve vessel occlusion more rapidly than stainless steel electrodes [22]. However, a comparison of platinum and stainless steel anodes showed that bipolar and monopolar platinum electrodes, but not stainless steel, caused localized perforation of the vessels [23] (Fig. 5). At present we have not found a satisfactory replacement for the standard unipolar stainless steel guidewire anode.

Recent work indicates that the intimal damage produced by the anode is not caused by thermal injury but is probably related to a marked decrease in pH at the electrode tip [16]. Since a greater decrease in pH at the anode tip is found with platinum than with stainless steel, this may explain why platinum anodes produced vessel perforation and stainless steel anodes did not.

During the past year, we compared two sizes and positions of anodes (0.025 inch versus 0.035 inch in diameter; placing the anodes out of the insulating catheter touching the vessel wall versus not touching the vessel wall). Comparisons were also made between two sizes of cathodes (1 × 1 cm versus 9 × 5 cm) as well as positioning the cathode directly over the anode versus moving the cathode away from the anode [15]. Changes in anode size and cathode size and position did not influence the extent of occlusion produced by TCEC, though, as was expected, high voltages were required to maintain a constant current with small anodes and cathodes. A more complete occlusion, however, was produced when the anode was in contact with the vessel wall than when it was not.

Increasing the current from 15 to 30 ma does not produce significantly faster or more complete occlusion [3]. However, 15 ma produces significantly better thrombus formation and vessel occlusion than either 5 or 10 ma [31].

In the early experiments, skin burns, similar to those reported by Leeming and coworkers [18], were noted at the site of the cathode when metallic needles were used for the negative ground [14]. Such burns have also occurred when a metal ground plate was used as the cathode (Fig. 6) [14]. However, protecting the skin from the metal ground plate with a highly lubricated sponge eliminates this problem [14, 22].

[1]   Hewlett-Packard, Palo Alto, California, USA, model 61816
[2]   American Hospital Supply, McGraw Park, Illinois, USA, Electrosurgical Pad No. 65418
[3]   John Fluke, Seattle, Washington, USA, 8,000 A

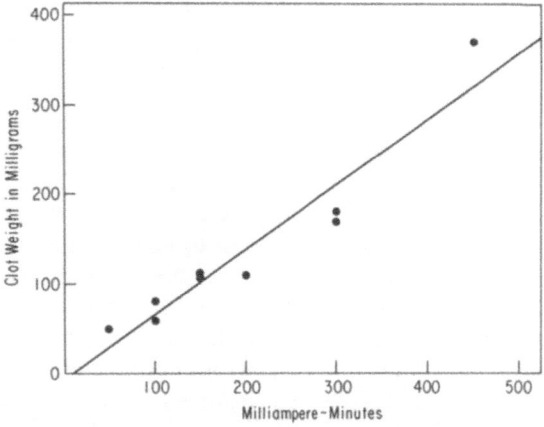

Fig. 2. Relationship of clot weight and milliampere-minutes. Line filled by linear regression using the method of least squares. $Y = 0.73X - 8.38$ ($r = 0.95$) (Reprinted with permission from [12].)

Clinical Trial (Figs. 7, 8, and 9)

We have used TCEC for vessel occlusion in combination with embolization in six patients in whom other interventional or surgical techniques were considered dangerous or unfeasible [20, 22, 34]. The six cases are summarized in the Table.

In combination with embolization with Gelfoam or Ivalon or both, TCEC was effective in decreasing or obliterating the blood supply to all lesions in these six patients. In seven of 17 vessels, a second application of TCEC was required to occlude the artery. Generally, these were larger vessels of 4–5 mm diameter. The time necessary for complete vessel occlusion ranged from six to 60 minutes (mean, 38 minutes). The voltage across the patient ranged from 9 to 40 V

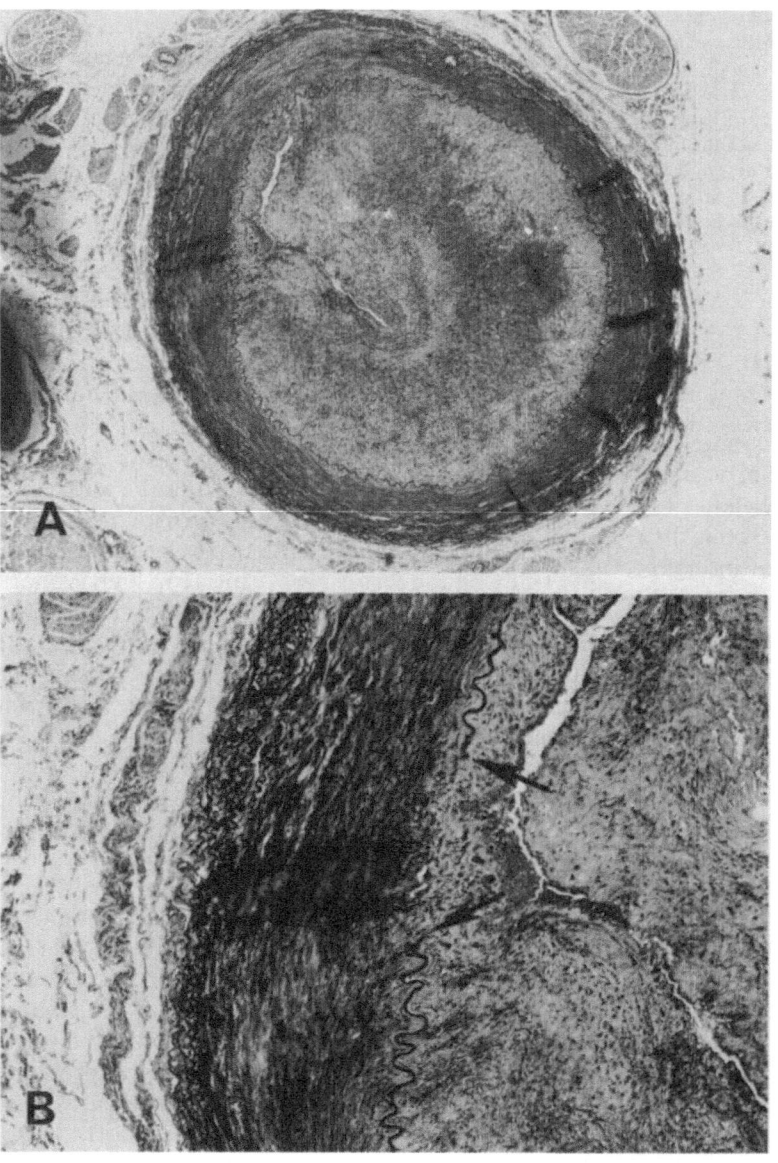

Fig. 3A and B. Microscopic section ($27 \times$) and magnification view of thrombosed splenic artery two months after coagulation. Vessel wall is intact but the internal elastic membrane is disrupted (*arrows*). Clot is firmly attached to the area of intimal destruction. (Reprinted with permission from [12].)

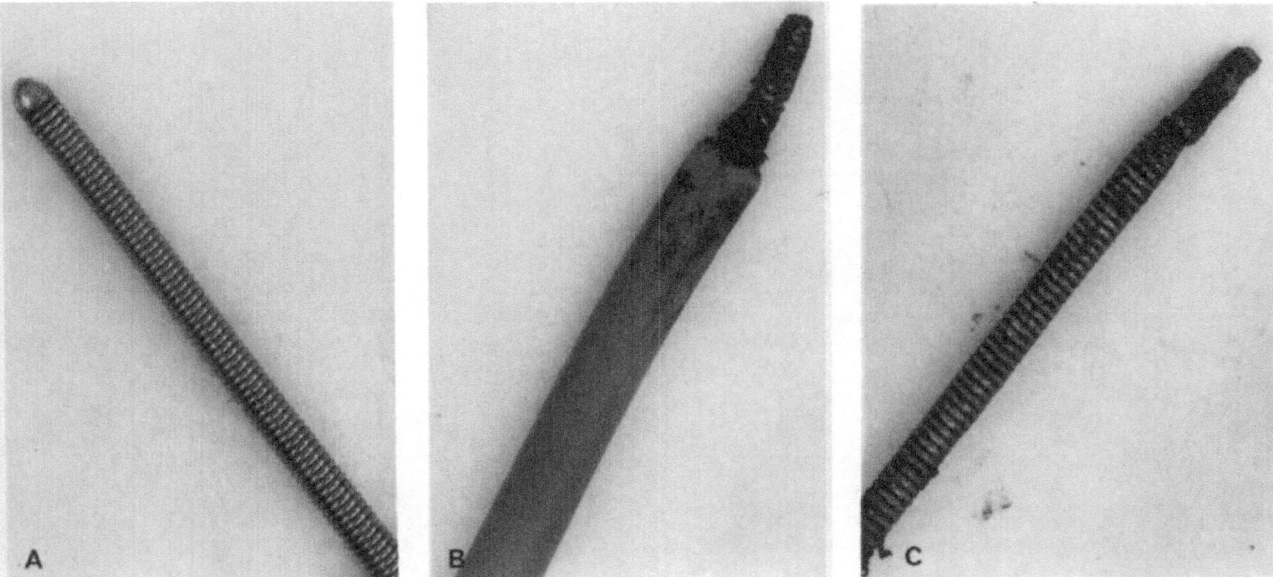

Fig. 4A–C. A Tip of guidewire before TCEC. **B** Guidewire protruding from catheter after 25 minutes of TCEC. **C** Tip of guidewire after 25 minutes of TCEC. Note destruction of wire due to electrolysis.

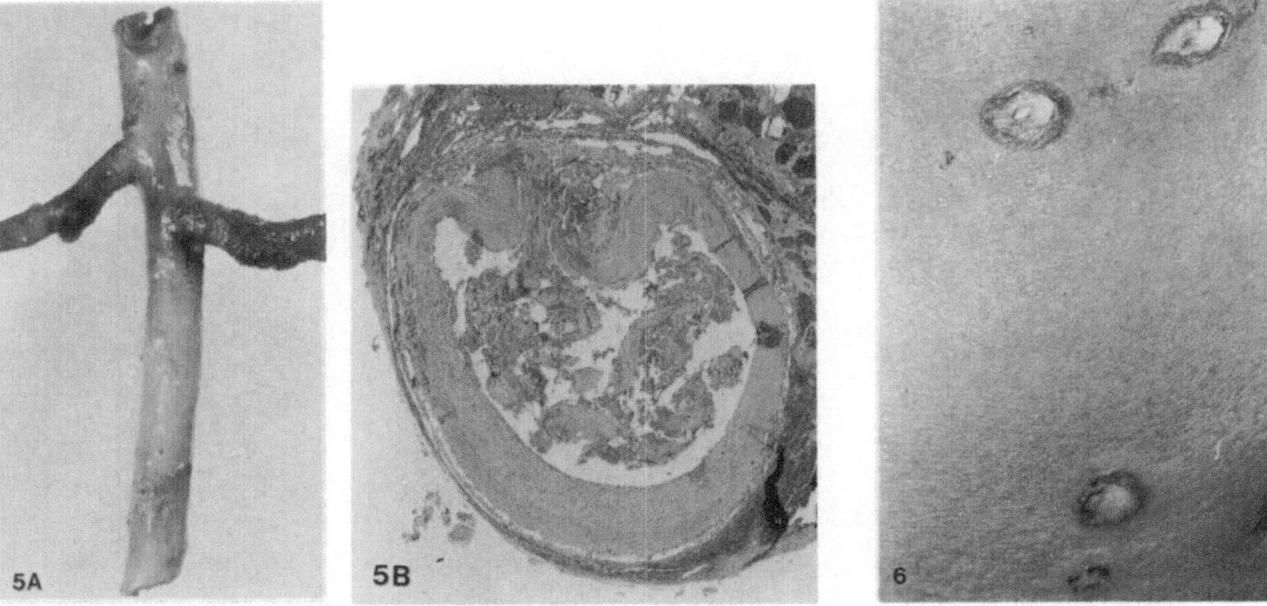

Fig. 5A and B. A Aorta with attached right and left renal arteries. Note evidence of vessel perforation on left and thrombus in right renal artery without evidence of perforation. **B** Cross-section of left renal artery (27×) showing perforation of vessel wall and lack of vessel occlusion. (Reprinted with permission from [12].)

Fig. 6. Skin burns after the use of metallic ground plate. (Reprinted with permission from [22].)

and in general tended to rise 20–50% during the procedure. However, we were not able to tell at exactly what voltage vessels became occluded.

In four of the six patients, the tip of the anode broke off and remained in the area of the thrombosis (Fig. 8). This generally occurred when TCEC had been performed for more than 25 minutes. As far as we know, this did not lead to any side effects.

In general, all patients tolerated the procedure well. There were no neurologic changes. While all the patients had varying degrees of pain for up to three days following TCEC, the only complications were small skin burns in case 3 (Fig. 6) and a small area of necrosis of the upper lip in case 6. The skin

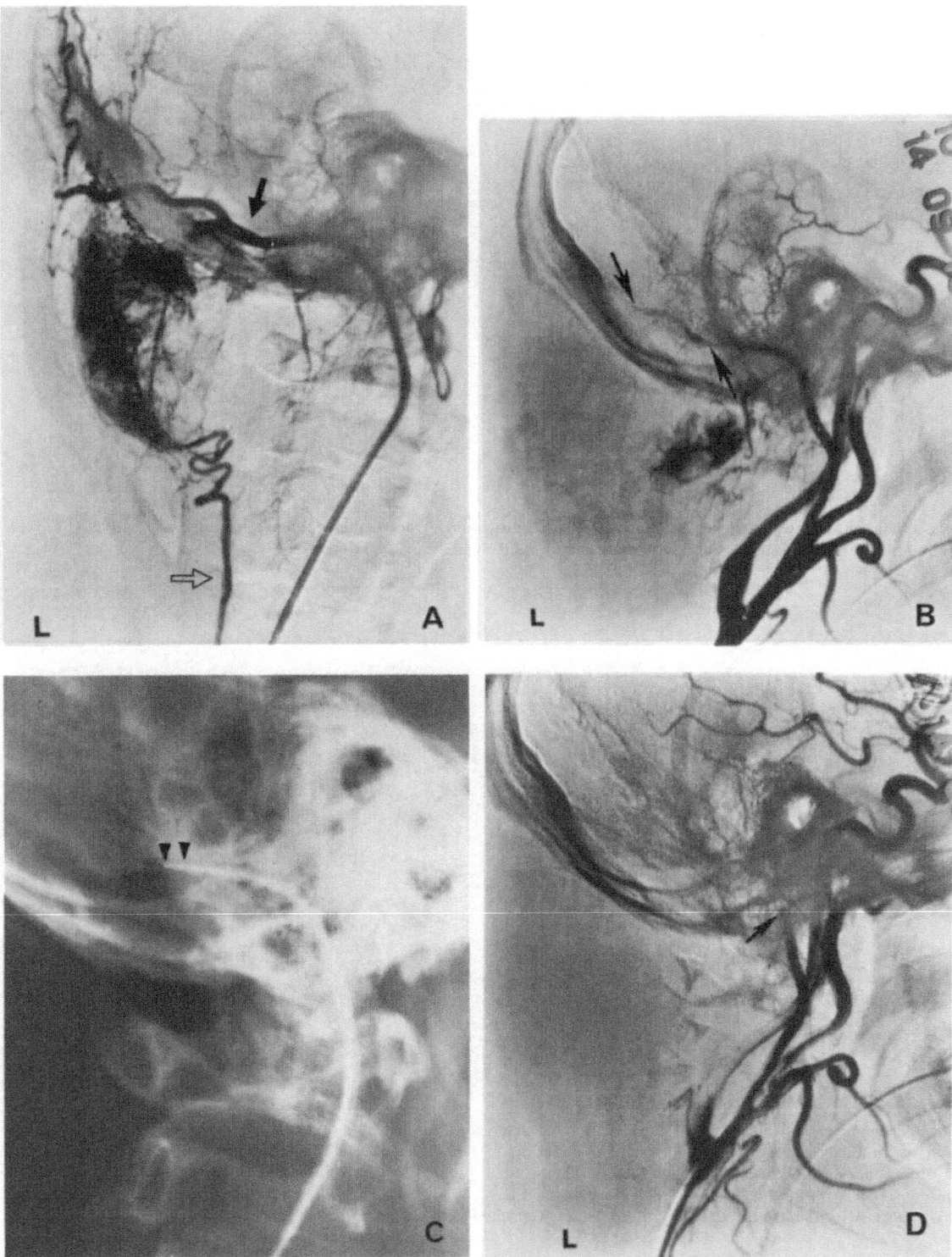

Fig. 7 A–D. A Preliminary angiogram showing vascular supply of tumor. *Open arrow:* ascending cervical artery. *Closed arrow:* occipital artery. **B** Gelfoam emboli occluding distal branches of the occipital artery (*arrows*). **C** Catheter in place in left posterior occipital artery with guidewire electrode protruding 2 mm beyond tip (*arrows*). **D** Complete occlusion of the occipital artery (*arrow*) following electrocoagulation. Note the streaming effect in the carotid circulation on this late arterial phase angiogram. (Reprinted with permission from [22].)

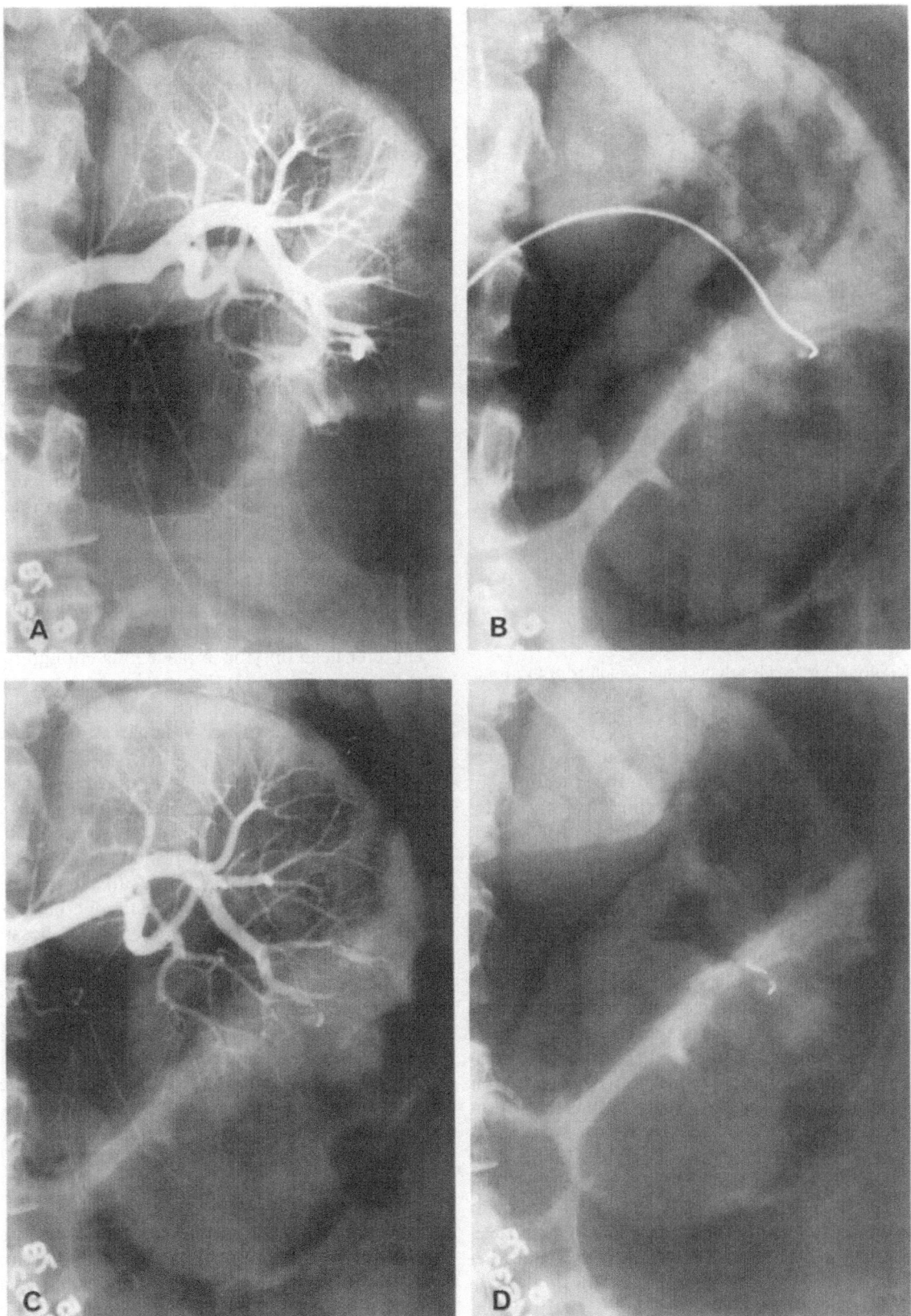

Fig. 8 A–E. A A left renal arteriogram of upper pole artery showing a large arteriovenous fistula. **B** Catheter and guidewire electrode in arteriovenous fistula during transcatheter electrocoagulation. **C** Arteriogram after transcatheter electrocoagulation demonstrates occlusion of arteriovenous fistula. **D** Plain film. Guidewire tips remain in thrombus. (Reprinted with permission from [20].) **E** see next page.

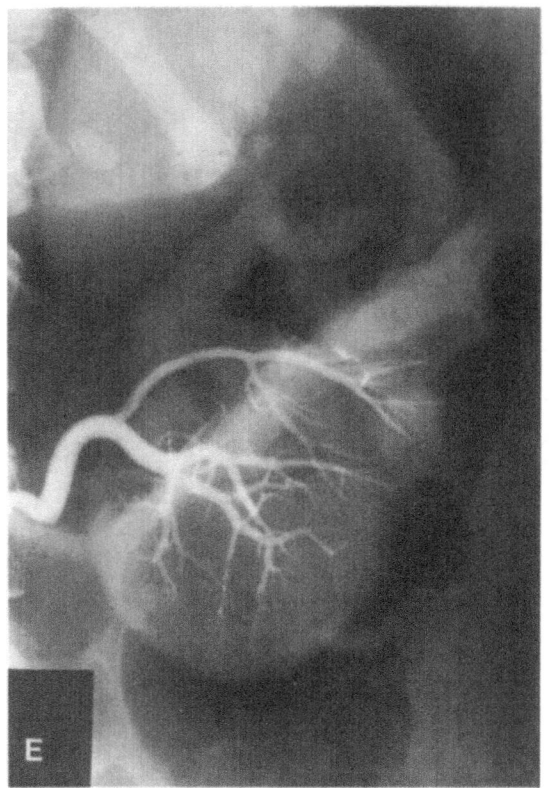

Fig. 8E. Normal lower pole arteriogram. (Reprinted with permission from [20].)

burns occurred when a metal bovie plate was inadvertently used to improve the ground connection. In this instance small (3–4 mm) alkaline skin burns developed within five minutes due to the hydrolysis [18, 22]. In all other cases, we were able to avoid such burns by protecting the skin from the metal ground plate with a highly lubricated sponge.

Although the electrocardiogram QRS complex is distorted by the TCEC current, we were still able to monitor a normal sinus rhythm, and the QRS complex returned to normal immediately upon discontinuing the TCEC current. An electroencephalogram, which was performed in two patients, was also distorted during TCEC but returned to normal after the procedure in a similar fashion to the electrocardiogram.

In the five cases in which vessels in the head or neck or both were involved, TCEC was carried out under general anesthesia (Figs. 7 and 9). The remaining patient (case 4) had a post-renal biopsy arteriovenous fistula and underwent TCEC with local anesthesia (Fig. 8). Initially she complained of flank pain when the current exceeded 7 ma, but after five minutes we were able to raise the current to 15 ma without additional discomfort. During a second application of TCEC, she had pain for five minutes at 10 ma

and then no pain when the current was raised to 15 ma. She did not complain of any symptoms from the cathode on her lower leg.

Case 6 was restudied six months after TCEC. The vessels were still occluded but collateral circulation had developed to supply the large facial arteriovenous malformation (Fig. 9).

Discussion

During the past 10 years, angiographers have introduced various drugs, balloons, and other materials through catheters to treat a variety of vascular lesions. All these methods have inherent problems, not only due to technical factors but also because of the potential for serious side effects, particularly occlusion of nontarget vessels. If precise, permanent vessel occlusions could be produced using electrical current, this might prove more advantageous in certain cases than methods presently employed.

The potential advantages of TCEC over other methods of vessel occlusion are: (1) the site of occlusion can be accurately determined and controlled by positioning the tip of the anode. (2) the angiographic catheter need only be in place long enough to occlude the target vessel, (3) the occlusion is permanent (at least up to three months), and (4) the technique is effective in the presence of heparinization and thrombocytopenia.

Potential disadvantages and problems with TCEC are: (1) it may be impossible to place the anode at the exact site of desired vessel occlusion, (2) up to an hour may be needed to occlude large vessels (larger than 5 mm in diameter), (3) a satisfactory anode has not been developed, (4) the technique has not shown consistent results, and (5) there is a possibility of downstream embolization.

In patients with arteriovenous malformations or hypervascular tumors, TCEC would not be effective as the sole method of interventional therapy, since more peripheral occlusion is required. However, after the distal vascular abnormality is obliterated (with emboli or tissue adhesives), TCEC could be helpful in such cases in occluding the more proximal vessels and could reduce the potential for reflux of emboli into nontarget organs. Mullan [23] and several Japanese investigators [1, 17, 37] have even used transarterial dc electrocoagulation to occlude intracranial arteriovenous lesions. All the disadvantages of TCEC, except the lack of an ideal anode, are also found with all the transcatheter techniques used for vessel occlusion.

The ideal TCEC system should: allow precise localization of vessel occlusion without risk of perfora-

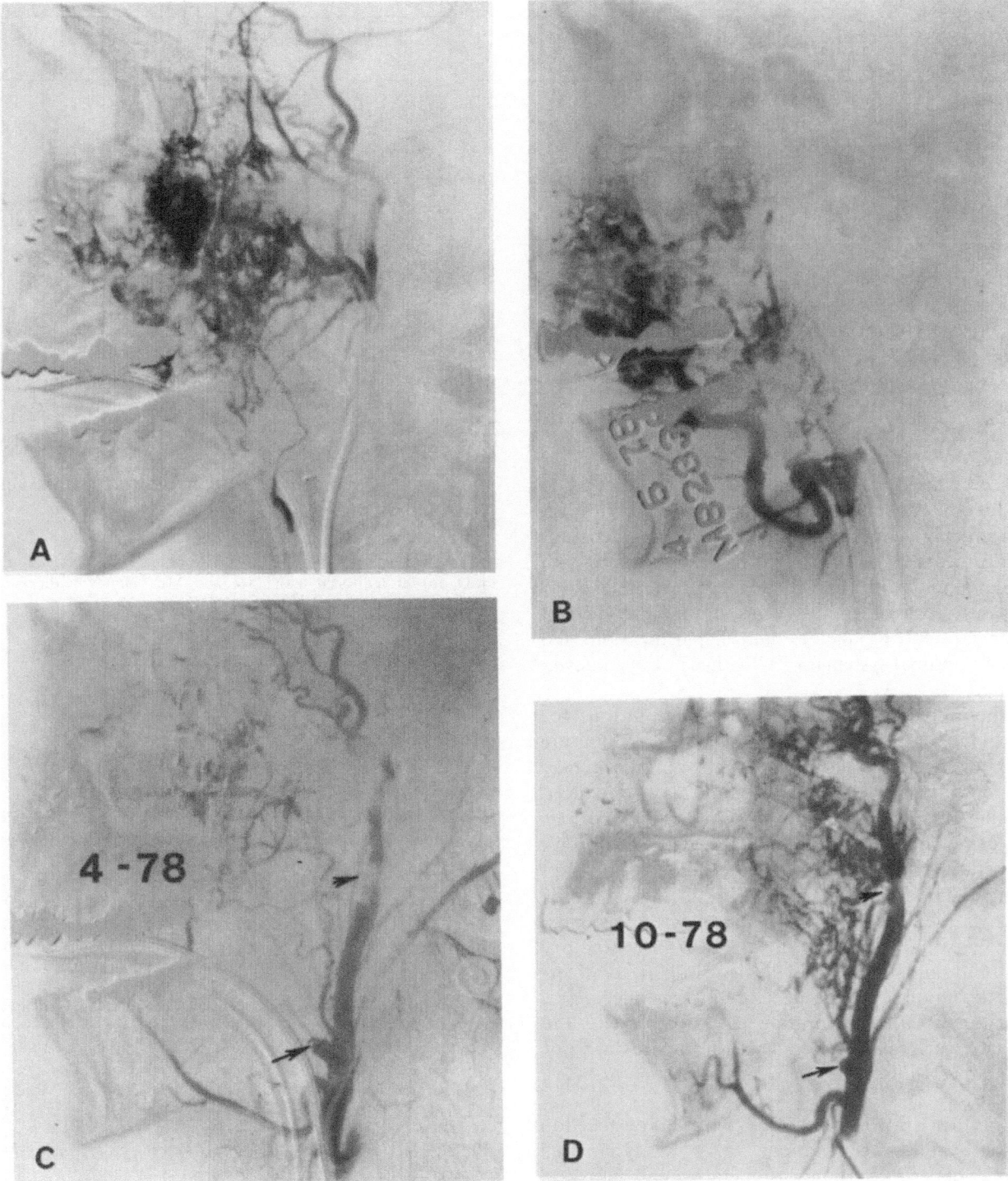

Fig. 9 A–D. A Subtraction radiograph, selective right internal maxillary angiogram, showing a large facial hemangioma. **B** Subtraction radiograph, selective right facial angiogram, showing a large facial hemangioma. **C** External carotid angiogram, showing complete occlusion of the origin of the internal maxillary (*arowhead*) and facial (*arrow*) arteries after TCEC. **D** Selective right external carotid angiogram six months after TCEC, showing complete occlusion of the internal maxillary (*arrowhead*) and facial (*arrow*) arteries. Note the extensive parasitic circulation supplying the large facial hemangioma. (Reprinted with permission from [34].)

Table. Summary of six cases in which transcatheter electrocoagulation was employed for vessel occlusion

Case	Diagnosis	No. vessels	No. attempts	Time (min)	Voltage (volts)	Comment
1	Massive venous hemangioma, face	8	10	25–60	16–40	Wire fragments in thrombosis; reduced size of mass
2	Bleeding carcinoma of the tongue	3	4	6–35	12–22	Controlled bleeding
3	Malignant paraganglioma	2	3	20–33	9–12	Excellent occlusion; good surgical results; skin burns.
4	Bleeding biopsy, renal arteriovenous fistula	1	2	60	16–20	Pain above 7 ma first 5 min; wire fragments in thrombosis; controlled hemorrhage
5	Hemagioma, left arm	1	2	60	16–40	Wire fragments in thrombosis; reduction in blood supply to mass.
6	Cavernous hemangioma, face	2	3	30–60	18–30	Reduced blood supply significantly; small area necrosis upper lip.

tion; be consistent, requiring only a few seconds to occlude the vessel; be painless; and carry no risk of producing ventricular fibrillation. It would be advantageous to be able to perform the procedure with standard guidewires and angiographic catheters. Finally, the technique must work in the presence of abnormal clotting factors and heparinization. To date, an optimal system for TCEC has not been developed.

There are a number of theoretical solutions for improving and further developing TCEC. A limiting factor in the technique is the length of time it may take to occlude large vessels. The time may be reduced by using alternating current (ac). Gold and coworkers [10], using ac from a surgical electrocoagulation unit via a standard steel guidewire to occlude vessels supplying a large false aneurysm in the head of the pancreas, achieved occlusion in only five seconds. However, Phillips found ac TCEC unsatisfactory in rabbits and dogs since it was difficult to determine the amount of current needed to produce vessel occlusion without perforation [24]. At present, the standard surgical electrocoagulation devices are not adequately calibrated, even for experimental work with ac.

Another drawback of TCEC with dc, destruction of the stainless steel anode, may be eliminated through experimentation with metals other than steel and platinum. Further evaluation of the possible mechanisms of TCEC may also provide new insights that could lead to the development of a more satisfactory system.

Although TCEC has been used safely in six patients, we do not feel that the technique, in its present form, is ready for wide clinical usage. If the method can be refined, it should, however, become a valuable addition to the techniques available to the interventional angiographer.

Acknowledgements. The authors wish to thank Laurence Hedlund, Ph.D. for his editorial assistance and Mrs. Nancy Holmes for her assistance in the preparation of the manuscript.

References

1. Araki, C., Handa, H., Yoshida, K.: Electrically induced thrombosis for the treatment of intracranial aneurysms and angiomas. Excerpta Medica International Congress Series 110:651–654, 1965
2. Athanasoulis, C.A., Baum, S., Waltman, A.A., Ring, E.J., Imbembo, A., Vander Salm, T.J.: Control of acute gastric mucosal hemorrhage. N. Engl. J. Med. 290:597–603, 1974
3. Baker, R., Hirschfeld, B., Pizzo, S., Thompson, W.M.: The effect of increasing current for transcatheter electrocoagulation (TCEC). Invest. Radiol. (in press)
4. Bookstein, J.J., Chlosta, E.M., Foley, D., Walter, J.F.: Transcatheter hemostasis of gastrointestinal bleeding using modified autogenous clot. Radiology 113:277–285, 1974
5. Bookstein, J.J., Goldstein, H.M.: Successful management of postbiopsy arteriovenous fistula with selective arterial embolization. Radiology 109:535–536, 1973
6. Carey, L.S., Grace, D.M.: The brisk bleed: Control by arterial catheterization and Gelfoam plug. J. Can. Assoc. Radiol. 25:113–115, 1974
7. Diulzio, V., Curri, G., Capestro, F., Boccanelli, A., Renzi, R.: Electrolytic phenomena and massive gas generation around pacemaker electrodes. Eur. J. Cardiol. 3:297, 1975
8. Dymond, A.M.: Characteristics of the metal tissue interfaced of stimulation electrodes. IEEE Trans. Biomed. Eng. 23:274–280, 1976
9. Eisenberg, H., Steer, J.L.: The nonoperative treatment of massive pyloroduodenal hemorrhage by retracted autologous clot embolization. Surgery 79:414–421, 1976
10. Gold, R.E., Blair, D.C., Finlay, J.D., Johnston, D.W.B.: Transarterial electrocoagulation therapy of a pseudoaneurysm in the head of the pancreas. Am. J. Roentgenol. 125:422–426, 1975

11. Goldman, M.L., Freeny, P.C., Tallman, J.M., Galambos, J.T., Bradley, E.L., Salom, A., Oen, K.-T., Gordon, I.J., Mennemeyer, R.: Transcatheter vascular occlusion therapy with isobutyl 2-cyanoacrylate (Bucrylate) for control of massive upper gastrointestinal bleeding. Radiology 129:41–49, 1978

12. Goldstein, H.M., Wallace, S., Anderson, J.H., Bree, R.L., Gianturco, C.: Transcatheter occlusion of abdominal tumors. Radiology 120:539–545, 1976

13. Gomes, A.S., Rysauy, J.A., Spadaccini, C.A., Probst, P., D'Souza, V., Amplatz, K.: The use of the bristle brush for transcatheter embolization. Radiology 129:345–350, 1978

14. Greatbatch, W., Piersma, B., Shannon, F.D., Calhoon, S.W.: Polarization phenomena relating to physiological electrodes. Advances in cardiac pacemakers. Ann. N.Y. Acad. Sci. 167:722–744, 1969

15. Hirschfeld, B.J., Clark, H.C., Thompson, W.M.: The effect of temperature and pH in transcatheter electrocoagulation (TCEC). Invest. Radiol. (in press)

16. Hirschfeld, B., McAlister, D.S., Lowther, D., Jackson, D.C., Pizzo, S., Thompson, W.M.: An evaluation of size and position of the anode and cathode during transcatheter electrocoagulation (TCEC). Invest. Radiol. 14:387, 1979

17. Hosobuchi, Y.: Electrothrombosis of carotid-cavernous fistula. J. Neurosurg. 42:76–85, 1975

18. Leeming, M.N., Ray, C., Jr., Howland, W.S.: Low voltage, direct current burns. JAMA 214:1681–1684, 1970

19. Loucks, R.B., Weinberg, H., Smith, M.: The erosion of electrodes by small currents. Electroencephalogr. Clin. Neurophysiol. 11:823, 1959

20. McAlister, D.S., Johnsrude, I.S., Miller, M.D., Clapp, J., Thompson, W.M.: Occlusion of an acquired renal arteriovenous fistula with transcatheter electrocoagulation: A case report. Am. J. Roentgenol. 132:998–1000, 1979

21. Miller, F.J., Rankin, R.S., Gliedman, J.B.: Experimental internal iliac artery embolization: Evaluation of low viscosity silicone rubber isobutyl 2-cyanoacrylate, and carbon microspheres. Radiology 129:51–58, 1978

22. Miller, M.D., Johnsrude, I.S., Limberakis, A.J., Jackson, B.C., Pizzo, S., Thompson, W.M.: Clinical use of transcatheter electrocoagulation. Radiology 129:211–214, 1978

23. Mullan, S.: Experiences with surgical thrombosis of intracranial berry aneurysms and carotid cavernous fistulas. J. Neurosurg. 41:657–670, 1974

24. Phillips, J.F.: Transcatheter electrocoagulation of blood vessels. Invest. Radiol. 8:295–304, 1973

25. Phillips, J.F., Robinson, A.E., Johnsrude, I.S., Jackson, D.C.: Experimental closure of arteriovenous fistulae by transcatheter electrocoagulation. Radiology 115:319–321, 1975

26. Rösch, J., Dotter, C.T., Brown, M.J.: Selective arterial embolization. A new method for control of acute gastrointestinal bleeding. Radiology 102:202–206, 1972

27. Rowley, B.A.: Electrolysis – a factor in cardiac pacemaker electrode failure. IEEE Trans. Biomed Electr. 10:176, 1963

28. Sawyer, P.N., Pate, J.W.: Bio-electrical phenomena as an etiologic factor in intravascular thrombosis. Am. J. Physiol. 175:103–107, 1973

29. Serbienko, F.A.: Balloon catheterization and occlusion of major cerebral vessels. J. Neurosurg 41:125–145, 1974

30. Tadavarthy, S.M., Moller, J.H., Amplatz, K.: Polyvinyl alcohol (Ivalon): A new embolic material. Am. J. Roentgenol. 125:609–616, 1975

31. Thompson, W.M., Pizzo, S.V., Jackson, D.C., Johnsrude, I.S.: Transcatheter electrocoagulation: A therapeutic angiographic technique for vessel occlusion. Invest. Radiol. 12:146–153, 1977

32. Thompson, W.M., Pizzo, S., Jackson, D.C., Johnsrude, I.S.: The effect of drug induced thrombocytopenia on direct current transcatheter electrocoagulation. Radiology 124:831–833, 1977

33. Thompson, W.M., McAlister, S., Miller, M., Pizzo, S.V., Jackson, D.C., Johnsrude, I.S.: Transcatheter electrocoagulation: An experimental evaluation of the anode. Invest Radiol. 14:41–47, 1979

34. Thompson, W.M., Johnsrude, I.S., Jackson, D.C., McAlister, S., Miller, M.D., Pizzo, S.V.: Vessel occlusion with transcatheter electroagulation: An initial clinical experience. Radiology 133:335–340, 1979

35. Wallace, S., Gianturco, C., Anderson, J.H., Goldstein, H.M., Davis, L.J., Bree, R.L.: Therapeutic vascular occlusion utilizing steel coil technique: Clinical applications. Am. J. Roentgenol. 127:381–387, 1976

36. White, R.I., Kaufmann, S.L., Barth, K.H., DeCaprio, V., Strandberg, J.D.: Embolotherapy with detachable silicone balloons: Technique and clinical results. Radiology 131:619–627, 1979

37. Yoneda, S., Matsuda, M., Shimizu, Y., Goto, H., Handa, H., Ogawa, Y.: Electrothrombosis of arteriovenous malformation. Neurol. Med. Chir. 17:19–28, 1977

Comment

Vessel Occlusion with Transcatheter Electrocoagulation: Negative Results

Kurt Amplatz

Department of Radiology, University Hospitals, University of Minnesota, Minneapolis, Minnesota, USA

Vessel occlusion by transcatheter electrocoagulation (TCEC) is an ingenious technique, which has the ma-

Address reprint requests to: K. Amplatz, M.D., Department of Radiology, University Hospitals, University of Minnesota, 420 Delaware Street S.E., Minneapolis, MN 55455, USA

jor advantage of achieving selective occlusion of arteries through the superselective placement of an electrode in peripheral branches. The technique does not depend on blood flow, and embolization of non-target vessels and other organs can be avoided. The technique also has the advantage of producing arterial occlusion in cases where the catheter cannot be advanced deeply enough into the feeding artery to allow safe embolization. As we all know, it is usually simpler to advance guidewires rather than catheters, which commonly do not follow the introduced guidewire. Another advantage appears to be the permanency of the vascular occlusion, which has been reported as persisting up to four months. However, since blood clots lyse in a short period of time, it is difficult to understand why the thrombi created by electrocoagulation behave differently from clots formed by spontaneous coagulation.

TCEC also has numerous disadvantages:

1. Preliminary in vitro experiments performed in our laboratory using the Thompson and Johnsrude electrocoagulation technique showed extremely slow clot formation. Although the authors demonstrate a fairly straight relationship between clot weight in milligrams and milliampere-minutes, this relationship may vary from one animal to the next. In our limited experience the formation of clots was indeed so variable and inconsistent that our experiments did not extend beyond in vitro pilot studies.

2. The technique does not lend itself to occlusion of larger arteries. Since the formed clots will be carried to the periphery in such cases, there is no advantage in forming blood clots by electrocoagulation over injecting preformed clots or synthetic materials.

3. The operator has no control over the size of formed emboli, and consequently the technique cannot be used to obliterate larger arteriovenous malformations.

4. Complete obliteration of larger arteries may be extremely time-consuming, requiring up to one hour of current application. This is a distinct disad-

vantage in the treatment of bleeding patients who may require immediate help.

5. It is most disturbing that the authors had to use a combination of particulate matter embolization and electrocoagulation in most cases. One wonders why electrocoagulation alone was not adequate.

6. Apparently the system is not flushed during the coagulation procedure, and consequently the progress of the vascular occlusion cannot be checked by test injections. The electrode wire also must be removed before the injection of contrast medium can be made. This system could be improved by connecting the catheter to a Y-connector with a gasket allowing continuous flushing and test injections.

7. The tip of the electrode undergoes electrolysis to the extent that it may break off and remain in the patient. Apparently, when and where this breakage occurs cannot be determined with certainty. Electrolysis of the guidewire also introduces theoretically toxic heavy-metal ions, such as iron, nickel, chromium, and a small amount of manganese. Since experiments with platinum electrodes have failed, gold or iridium plating of the guidewire tip might perhaps be considered. As long as the electrode problem is not solved, widespread clinical application of the technique cannot be encouraged, and Federal Drug Administration approval may be difficult to obtain.

In summary, TCEC represents an interesting technique that allows the superselective occlusion of peripheral arteries without employing emboli. The numerous drawbacks of the technique in its present form preclude widespread clinical use, but the authors should be encouraged to continue their interesting research.

Reply

William M. Thompson and Irwin S. Johnsrude

We appreciate the critical comments by Dr. Amplatz. With any new technique there are always problems as well as advantages and disadvantages. Dr. Amplatz has very astutely addressed the practical benefits and many problems of transcatheter electrocoagulation.

We agree that it is difficult to understand why thrombosis with electrocoagulation produces a permanent occlusion. Perhaps the minor amount of intimal damage from electocoagulation produces permanent thrombosis. The end products of electrolysis of the anode may also play a role.

Dr. Amplatz found such variability and inconsistency with electrocoagulation that he did not move past in vitro pilot studies. As pointed out in our work, while there is some variability, one can occlude vessels 5–6 mm in size within one hour. We disagree with Dr. Amplatz's statement that the technique does not lend itself to occlusion of larger arteries since formed clots will be carried into the periphery. We have not had any significant downstream embolization with this technique. We certainly have no control over the size of the formed emboli but disagree with

Dr. Amplatz's statement that the technique cannot be used to obliterate larger arteriovenous malformations. We have shown in our clinical work that this technique may be used in conjunction with embolization to occlude even large AVM's.

The technique may be extremely time consuming, requiring up to one hour. This may be a distinct disadvantage in patients who are bleeding and require immediate help. To date, no one has had any experience with direct current electrocoagulation in these particular patients. In our experience, most patients with intestinal bleeding have feeding vessels less than 3–4 mm in size, which usually can be occluded in 15 to 30 minutes.

We are not sure why Dr. Amplatz was so disturbed that we used a combination of embolization of particulate matter and electrocoagulation in most cases since four of our six patients had large vascular lesions. Some authors have stated that it requires an extensive period of time to embolize these large lesions, and occlusion of larger feeding vessels may be problematic since there is a major risk of embolization of unwanted vessels. We feel the combination of embolization and electrocoagulation may provide successful occlusion of vascular lesions with a lower risk than embolization alone.

We appreciate Dr. Amplatz's comment concerning the improvement in the technique. We are evaluating a system for continuous flushing. To date, since we have used the smallest catheter possible, we have not had success flushing the catheter containing the anode during the procedure.

The fact that the electrode tip undergoes electrolysis and may break off and remain in the patient does not appear to be a major problem. All embolized synthetic material remains in the patient, and there is no evidence that these embolized materials are less toxic than steel wire. Certainly this wire is similar to the numerous surgical clips and staples that are used by surgeons. If the electrocoagulation is stopped at 20 or 25 minutes, the electrode tip rarely breaks. There is a theoretical objection that the electrolysis of the guidewire may introduce toxic heavy metal ions. We are in the process of evaluating these end products. We are also evaluating many metals to find a more satisfactory anode.

In summary, many of the objections to and disadvantages of the technique, as pointed out by Dr. Amplatz, have been recognized by us. We appreciate his candid comments and criticisms and also his encouragement in the continuation of our work. All currently used therapeutic embolic techniques have major disadvantages. Each carries the risk of producing occlusion of non-target vessels, and all introduce a foreign body into the arterial system with the exception of embolization with autologous clot, which has the disadvantage of rapid lysis. Theoretically, transcatheter electrocoagulation has major advantages over all of these methods. Further refinements and improvements must, however, be made before the technique will gain wide usage.

Current Status of Transcatheter Management of Neoplasms

Vincent P. Chuang and Sidney Wallace

Department of Diagnostic Radiology, The University of Texas System Cancer Center, M.D. Anderson Hospital and Tumor Institute, Houston, Texas, USA

Abstract. Transcatheter arterial infusion and arterial embolization are employed in the treatment of various neoplasms. In patients with carcinoma of the colon metastatic to the liver, the hepatic arterial infusion (HAI) of floxuridine and Mitomycin© produced a 55% partial response and a 12% complete response, as well as an improved median survival of 18 months. In metastatic breast carcinoma, a 30% response was achieved. In some cases, proximal embolization of aberrant hepatic arteries was performed to redistribute the hepatic flow to a single vessel to assist infusion of the entire liver using a single catheter. Devascularization by hepatic artery embolization has also been used to treat hepatic neoplasms. Arterial occlusion of renal carcinoma, followed after four to seven days by nephrectomy and hormonal therapy, produced a 36% response rate in 49 patients with distant metastases. In 14 patients with osteosarcoma treated with cis-diaminedichloroplatinum (CDDP) arterial infusion, a 57% response rate was achieved. Benign bone tumors were treated with arterial occlusion with a 60% response rate. Tumors of the pelvis were managed by bilateral internal iliac artery infusion using CDDP. In 21 patients with recurrent bladder carcinoma, control of pain and hematuria and prolonged survival were achieved.

Key words: Arterial infusion – Arterial embolization – Hepatic neoplasm – Renal carcinoma – Osteosarcoma – Bladder carcinoma – Interventional angiography.

The futility of existing therapy for certain neoplasms has stimulated exploration into interventional radio-logic techniques. Many interventional procedures that were initially performed out of desperation have now been incorporated into primary therapeutic management. Of the 100 angiographic examinations performed each month at M.D. Anderson Hospital and Tumor Institute (MDAH), about 60% are interventional. Although 10 to 15 arterial embolizations are performed each month, the percutaneous transcatheter intraarterial infusion of chemotherapeutic agents accounts for the majority of the interventional procedures. With the advent of superselective catheterization, newer chemotherapeutic agents, and a higher dose-time relationship, the intraarterial infusion technique has been resurrected in an attempt to improve the survival of patients with selected hepatic neoplasms. In addition, the use of intraarterial infusion has been extended to tumors at other sites, including the musculoskeletal system and the genitourinary tract.

Arterial embolization and occlusion have been effective in the treatment of renal carcinoma, primary and secondary hepatic neoplasms, and benign and malignant bone tumors. The indications for transcatheter embolization of neoplasms are: (1) to control hemorrhage; (2) preoperatively, to facilitate resection by decreasing blood loss and operating time; (3) to inhibit tumor growth; (4) to relieve pain; and perhaps (5) to stimulate an immune response to the ischemic neoplasm. These contributions and other potential applications of interventional radiology to the therapeutic management of patients with certain neoplastic diseases will be described.

Liver

The liver is the major organ most frequently involved by metastatic disease. Hepatic metastases rather than the primary neoplasms usually govern the course of

Address reprint requests to: V.P. Chuang, M.D., Department of Diagnostic Radiology, The University of Texas System Cancer Center, M.D. Anderson Hospital and Tumor Institute, Houston, TX 77030, USA

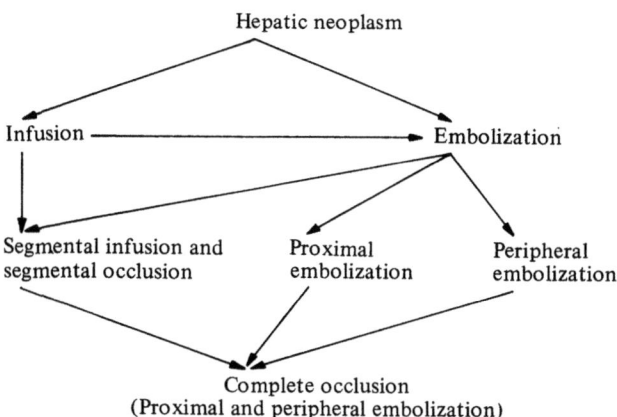

Fig. 1. Approach in cases with hepatic neoplasms.

the disease and the patient's survival. The median survival duration for patients with untreated liver metastases from carcinoma of the colon is 150 days; from carcinoma of the stomach, 60 days; and from carcinoma of the pancreas, 50 days [1]. In view of this ominous prognosis, an aggressive therapeutic approach is justified.

The transcatheter management of hepatic neoplasms, whether primary or secondary, includes arterial infusion and occlusion. Hepatic arterial infusion (HAI) of chemotherapeutic agents is a viable treatment alternative if the disease is localized in the liver, especially if systemic therapy has failed. The presence of aberrant vessels may necessitate redistribution of hepatic arterial supply by the intentional occlusion of certain vessels to allow optimal delivery of chemotherapeutic agents through a single artery. Peripheral embolization alone or in combination with central occlusion of the hepatic artery is frequently performed if the patient fails to respond to HAI or if effective drugs are not available. Our interventional angiographic approach to the liver is outlined in Figure 1. It should be stressed that if a hepatic neoplasm is localized to a resectable segment, then surgery is still the treatment of choice.

Hepatic Arterial Infusion

Patients with hepatic metastases from colorectal carcinoma have a median survival of five months (with a range as long as two years from the time of diagnosis); intravenous chemotherapy extends the median survival to one year. Liver metastases refractory to systemic chemotherapy may respond to HAI [2]. The rationale for HAI is based on the observation that most antitumor agents have a steep dose-response curve; that is, the higher the concentration of the drug, the greater the antitumor effect and the greater

ment alternative if the disease is localized in the liver, especially if systemic therapy has failed. The presence of aberrant vessels may necessitate redistribution of hepatic arterial supply by the intentional occlusion of certain vessels to allow optimal delivery of chetions while keeping the side effects to a minimum [4–6].

Currently, a combination of mitomycin C (MTC) and floxuridine (5-FUDR) is delivered by HAI to hepatic metastases from colorectal cancer. Both drugs are metabolized by the liver. The 5-FUDR was selected over 5-fluorouracil (5-FU) because of the higher extraction of 5-FUDR by the liver, which makes possible a shorter course of therapy (five days) [6].

Catheterization Technique. A high brachial or axillary infusion of chemotherapeutic agents. The catheter is fixed in place by the use of a plastic adhesive [1] covered by soft surgical tape [2]. To minimize thrombotic complications, 10,000–25,000 units per day of aqueous heparin are administered via HAI or intravenously is placed into the hepatic artery; from the femoral artery, a 65 cm (5 or 6.5 French) catheter is used. ment alternative if the disease is localized in the liver, especially if systemic therapy has failed. The presence of aberrant vessels may necessitate redistribution of hepatic arterial supply by the intentional occlusion of certain vessels to allow optimal delivery of chewhen technically feasible. With reversed (hepatopetal) flow in the gastroduodenal artery, which is seen more frequently with hypervascular metastases, placement of the catheter in the common hepatic artery is adequate. Superselective catheterization with placement in the desired hepatic vessel is accomplished in at least 90% of patients.

Infusion Technique. The catheter is connected to a pump (e.g., McGraw or Sigmamotor) for continuous infusion of chemotherapeutic agents. The catheter is fixed in place by the use of a plastic adhesive [1] covered by soft surgical tape [2]. To minimize thrombotic complications, 10,000–25,000 units per day of aqueous heparin are administered via HAI or intravenously (IV) to achieve and maintain a one and one-half-fold prolongation of the partial thromboplastin time (PTT). Heparin is incompatible with certain chemotherapeutic agents, such as adriamycin, and must therefore, be administered separately by IV while the adriamycin is being given by HAI. Aspirin, 650 mg, is dispensed orally twice a day beginning 24 hours before catheterization.

A conventional roentgenogram of the abdomen is taken daily to check the catheter position. In the event of catheter displacement during the treatment

---

[1] Op-Site, Smith & Nephew Inc., Lachine, Quebec, Canada
[2] Microfoam, 3M Company, St. Paul, MN 55101, USA

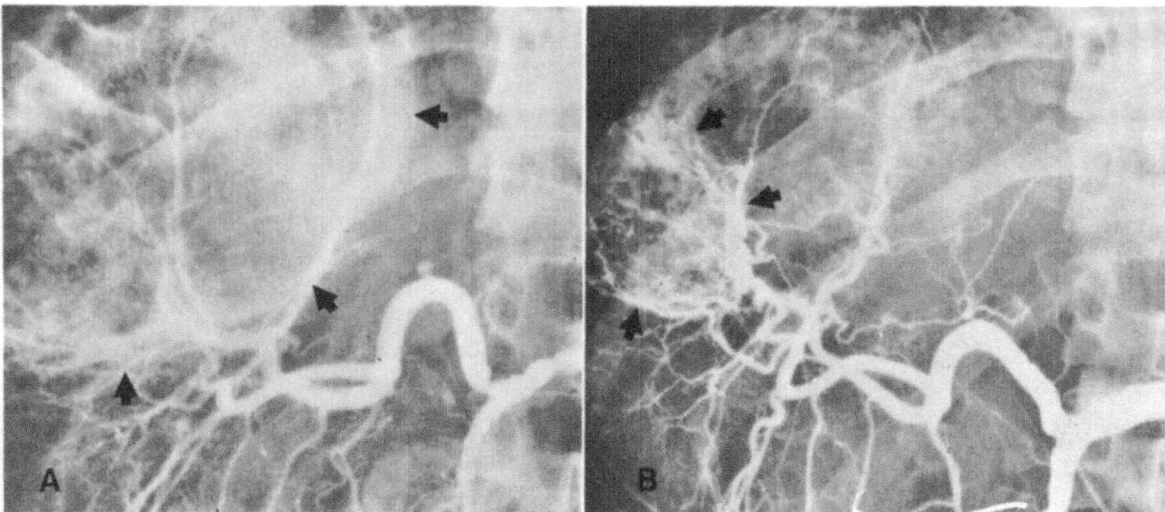

Fig. 2A and B. Carcinoma of colon with liver metastasis. **A** Hepatic arteriogram reveals a large conglomerated mass *(arrows)* in the right lobe. **B** After three courses of HAI, the mass *(arrows)* decreased to less than 25% of its original size.

course, the catheter is bathed with antiseptic solution, replaced, and secured. Antibiotics are then instituted prophylactically.

Selection of Drugs. Administration of MTC, 15 mg/ m², over a two-to-24 hour period and of 5-FUDR, 100 mg/m² per day, for a five-day continuous infusion is the present protocol for hepatic metastases from colorectal carcinoma [7]. Adriamycin, 60–75 mg/m² given over the course of five days in three pulses of 20–25 mg/m² each, is added to the protocol in cases with a primary hepatocellular neoplasm or metastases from a variety of other primary carcinomas. For metastases from breast carcinoma, soft tissue sarcomas, and melanoma, cis-diamminedichloroplatinum (CDDP), 120 mg/m², is infused over two hours [8]. Other agents have also been employed for HAI including 5-FU, cyclophosphamide, vincristine, and imidazole carboxamide. The treatment course is repeated every four to six weeks depending upon the patient's tolerance. Before the use of a new agent, its effects on the intima, especially its potential for causing vasculitis, with subsequent stenosis and/or occlusion, must be investigated in laboratory animals.

Results. Selective hepatic arteriography is performed before each infusion in order to delineate the vascular supply and its patency, to establish or document the diagnosis, and to evaluate the tumor response since the previous course of treatment. The tumor response is estimated by determining the change in the product of the two maximum perpendicular dimensions of a circumscribed lesion. Computed tomography and ultrasonography are used at times to assist in the evaluation. Tumor response is classified as CR (com-

plete response) and PR (partial response of 50% or greater). A case of partial response is illustrated in Figure 2.

Of the patients with colorectal carcinoma metastatic to the liver treated with at least three courses of 5-FUDR and MTC and followed up to two years, 55% experienced a partial response and 12% achieved a complete response. The median survival rate of patients in whom HAI was used as the first-line therapy was not significantly better than that of patients treated by the intravenous route. However, with HAI as a second line of therapy following the failure of intravenously administered chemotherapy, there was a significant improvement of survival from 12 months to 18 months with HAI. Among ten evaluable patients from a group of 14 with metastatic breast carcinoma confined to the liver and treated by HAI with CDDP, the response rate was 30% (CR 10%; PR 20%).

Comment. Improved results are necessary to warrant the increased risk and expense to the patient associated with the use of HAI. These will be pursued by means of: (1) meticulous and persistent efforts in selective catheter placement; (2) employment of higher drug concentrations over a shorter time interval; and (3) repeated hepatic arterial infusion. One patient received 17 treatment courses during his two-year-and-three-month survival, and several other patients were subjected to more than 10 courses.

The radiation exposure to the radiologist, the time and energy required, and the available radiographic facilities are serious limitations to the use of HAI. Because of these aspects of the treatment, HAI is limited to a cycle of three courses at monthly intervals and, for patients who respond, three additional

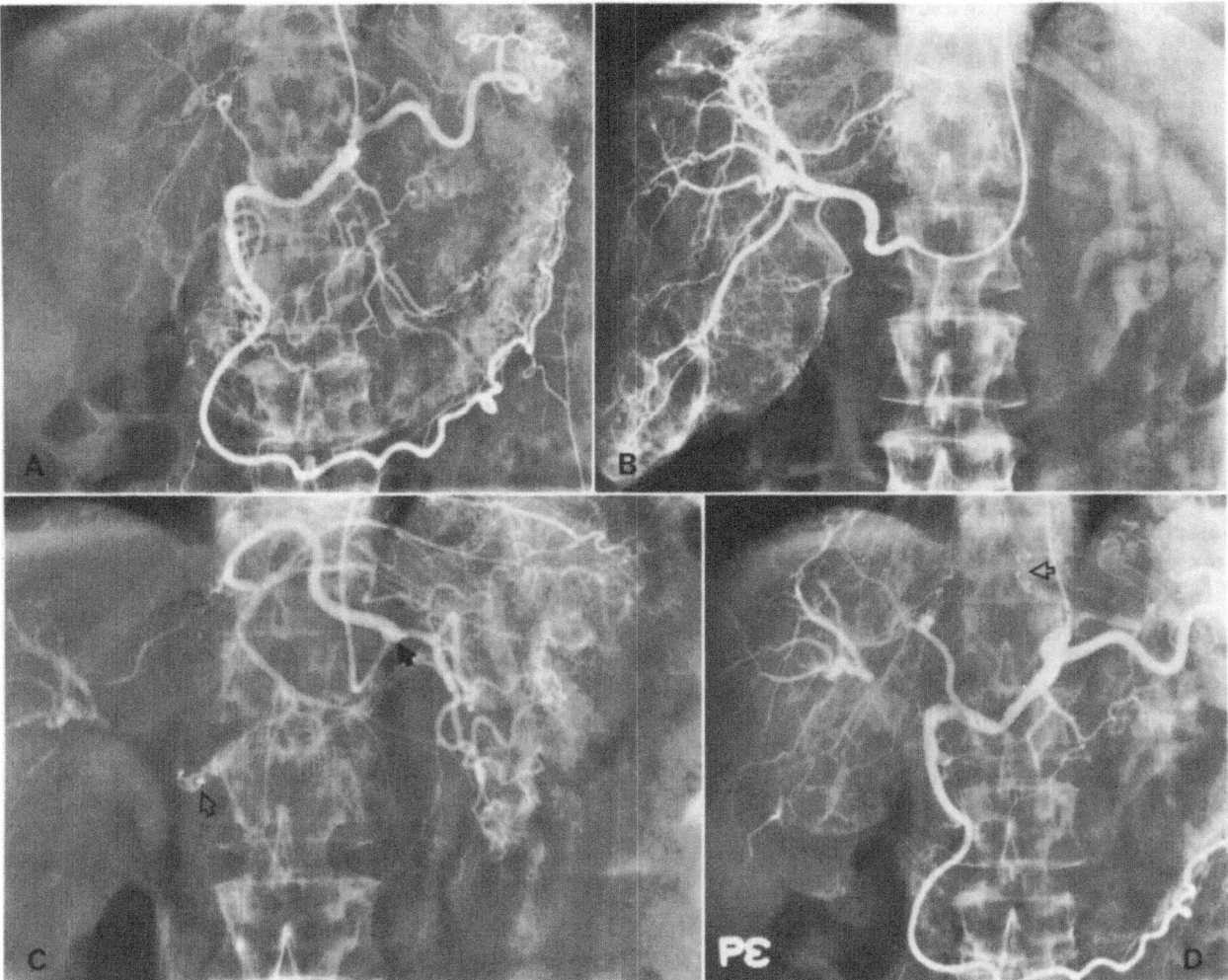

Fig. 3A–D. Redistribution of hepatic flow. Carcinoma of breast with liver metastasis. Michel's type IV hepatic artery anatomy. **A** Common hepatic arteriogram reveals a small mid-hepatic artery supplying the medial segment of the left lobe. **B** Accessory right hepatic artery from superior mesenteric artery supplies the right lobe. **C** Left hepatic artery, originating from left gastric artery, supplies the left lateral segment. The catheter tip *(closed arrow)* is at the junction of left gastric and left hepatic arteries. Note coil occlusion of the right hepatic artery *(open arrow)*. The catheter was advanced beyond left gastric artery, and the left hepatic artery was occluded with coils. **D** The catheter is repositioned at the common hepatic artery. Note instantaneous development of intrahepatic collaterals from the mid-hepatic artery to the right hepatic artery and the increase in size of the mid-hepatic artery. The collateral circulation to left hepatic artery is less prominent. Arrow denotes the coil in the occluded left hepatic artery.

courses. Failure by some patients to respond to HAI has led to an investigation of interventional alternatives, including hepatic artery embolization.

Redistribution of Hepatic Flow

An aberrant hepatic artery, which occurs in 50% of the general population, is a significant obstacle to HAI. A decrease in tumor size in one lobe with a simultaneous increase in the noninfused lobe has been repeatedly observed following HAI. The use of two catheters when necessary (one in the celiac hepatic artery and the other in the replaced hepatic artery

from the superior mesenteric artery) increases the time of the procedure, radiation exposure, and patient discomfort. Transcatheter occlusion of the aberrant hepatic artery has been performed to redistribute the hepatic arterial flow to a single vessel [9]. For example, in a patient with a Michel's type IV hepatic artery anatomy – branching of the right hepatic artery from the superior mesenteric artery, the left hepatic artery (lateral segment) from the left gastric artery, and the middle hepatic artery (medial segment of left hepatic) from the celiac or common hepatic artery – both the right and left hepatic arteries were occluded proximally using 5 French coils [10–12] (Fig. 3). The catheter was placed in the common hepatic artery to infuse the middle hepatic artery and the entire liver through intrahepatic collateral circulation.

Complications of HAI

Vascular trauma is associated both with superselective catheterization and with the introduction of a higher concentration of agents over a shorter infusion time. With vascular trauma there is a 17% incidence of occlusion and a 6% incidence of aneurysm. A greater experience in the technical aspects, careful drug administration and the achievement of adequate anticoagulation have minimized these complications.

Gastrointestinal Complications. The arterial blood supply to the stomach, duodenum, gallbladder, and pancreas also originates from the hepatic artery. Unavoidable infusion of the gastroduodenal and the right gastric arteries has resulted in dyspepsia in 11.6% of patients; some had documented gastritis, duodenitis, gastric and duodenal ulcers, cholecystitis and pancreatitis.

In approximately half the population, there is a proper hepatic artery; that is, the gastroduodenal artery arises midway between the origin of the common hepatic artery from the celiac artery and its division into the right and left hepatic arteries.. In a quarter of the population, the gastroduodenal artery arises either at the bifurcation of the common hepatic artery (i.e., as a trifurcation with the right and left hepatic arteries) or it arises distal to the hepatic bifurcation (i.e., directly from either the right or left hepatic arteries). In the remaining quarter, the gastroduodenal artery comes from replaced hepatic arteries or from other sources. Placement of the infusion catheter beyond the gastroduodenal artery will decrease the unintentional infusion of chemotherapeutic agents to the duodenum, stomach, and pancreas. Occasionally, the gastroduodenal artery has reversed (hepatopetal) flow, which allows safe placement of the catheter in the common hepatic artery. Occlusion of the gastroduodenal artery using a coil has been performed in selected patients who developed severe gastrointestinal symptoms.

The right gastric artery originates in the proper hepatic artery in 40% of the population and in the left hepatic artery in 41.5%. It is small (2 mm or less) and frequently unnoticed in a celiac arteriogram, though it can be identified in most selective hepatic arteriograms. In a series of 18 patients who experienced gastrointestinal symptoms following HAI, the majority of the symptoms could be attributed to the infusion of the right gastric artery with a high dose of chemotherapeutic agent over a short period of time.

Hepatic Occlusion

Primary and secondary hepatic neoplasms receive 90% of their blood supply from the hepatic artery, although the normal liver parenchyma has a dual supply, with 30% deriving from the hepatic artery and 70% from the portal vein. Following hepatic artery ligation, there is a 90% decrease in blood flow to the tumor and a 30–40% decrease in flow to the normal parenchyma [13]. Mori has reported selective destruction of the tumor without damage to the normal liver after ligation of the hepatic artery for metastatic gastric carcinoma [14]. The response to surgical ligation is temporary, partly because of the formation of collateral circulation. Collateral circulation may develop instantaneously following proximal occlusion of the hepatic artery for redistribution of hepatic flow (Fig. 3).

Devascularization of a hepatic neoplasm can be achieved percutaneously by combined peripheral embolization of particulate material (Gelfoam) and central occlusion with a stainless steel coil. This method can be used: (1) in patients with unresectable primary hepatic neoplasms; (2) preoperatively, to facilitate surgery of a resectable neoplasm; (3) in metastatic neoplasms that fail to respond to chemotherapy; (4) as the initial management of certain metastases usually refractory to chemotherapy; and (5) to control pain and/or hemorrhage from a hepatic neoplasm. Figure 4 illustrates the effects of repeated embolization of the hepatic artery with Gelfoam in a patient with an unresectable cholangiocarcinoma. The patient is still alive 4.5 years after the first embolization.

Kidney

Annually, approximately 15,000 Americans develop renal adenocarcinoma and 7,500 succumb to this disease. In 25–40% of cases, the patients present with metastases. With pulmonary metastases, chemotherapy and hormonal therapy yield a 25% and an 18% remission, respectively, but no prolongation of survival [15, 16]. Nephrectomy in patients with lung metastases does not significantly affect the median survival which is 5.4 months without nephrectomy and 7.9 months with nephrectomy. In contrast, nephrectomy may improve the median survival in patients with osseous metastases – the median survival is 10.6 months without nephrectomy versus 16 months with – but it has only proved effective in patients with solitary metastases [17].

At MDAH arterial occlusion of renal carcinoma was initially performed to facilitate the removal of hypervascular neoplasms. Subsequently, a protocol of infarction, nephrectomy, and hormonal therapy with medroxy-progesterone was designed for the man-

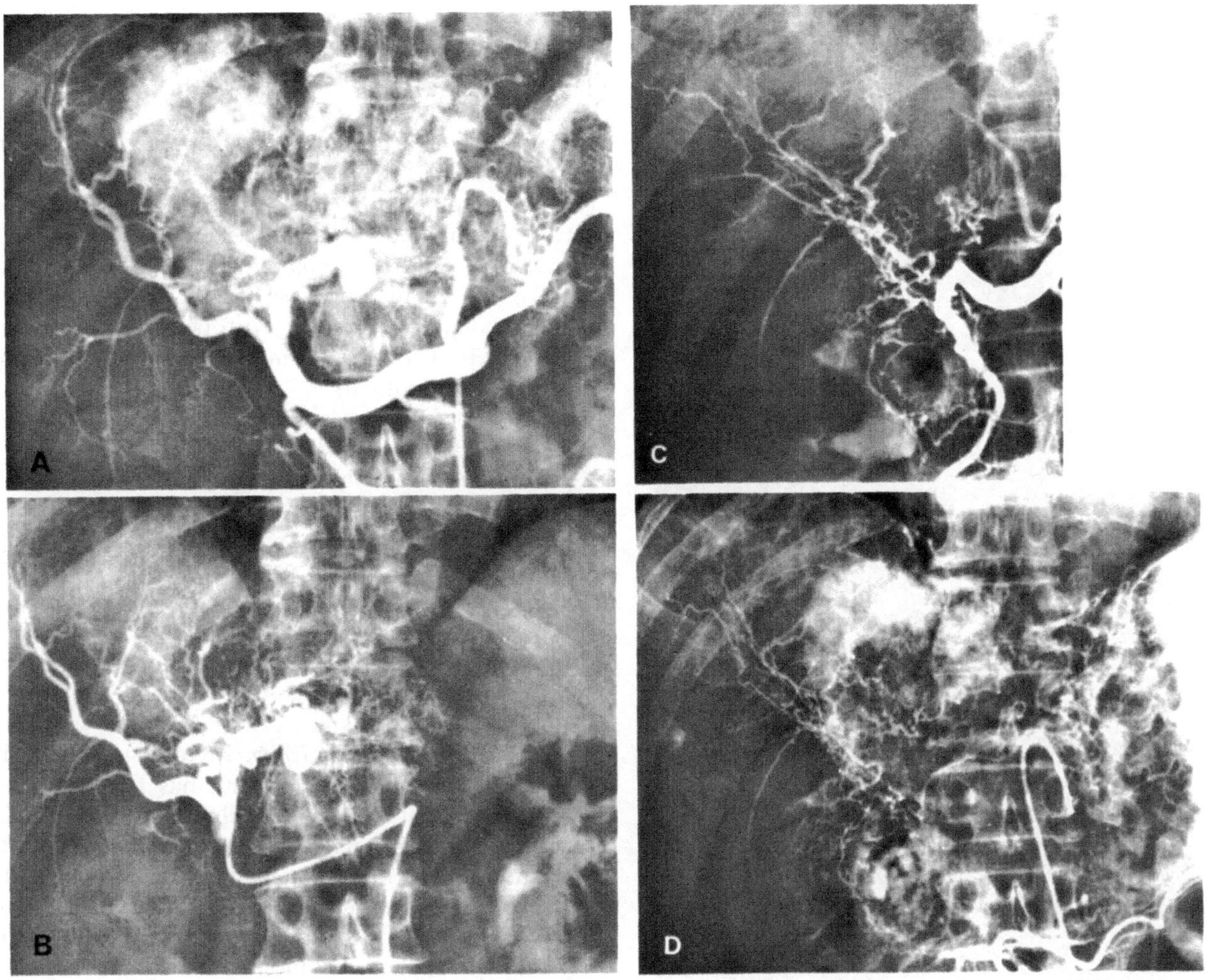

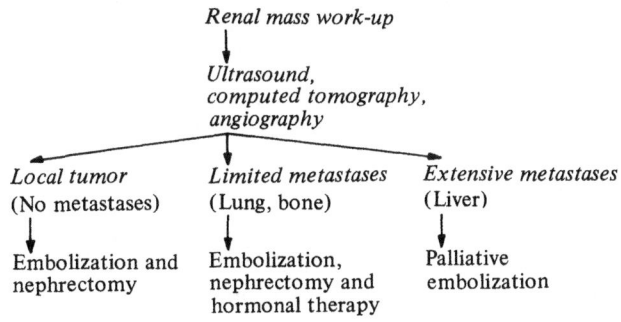

Fig. 4A–D. Cholangiocarcinoma of the liver. The mass was found to be unresectable in an exploratory laparotomy. **A** Celiac arteriogram shows a hypervascular mass predominantly in the left lobe. The left hepatic artery was selectively embolized with Gelfoam. **B** Follow-up hepatic arteriogram one week later reveals a significant decrease in tumor bulk and persistent occlusion in the periphery of the tumor along with the development of multiple collaterals near the center of the mass. The entire hepatic artery was completely embolized with Gelfoam, and three months after this second embolization, the proper hepatic artery was surgically ligated. **C** Follow-up arteriogram 14 months after first embolization demonstrates multiple collaterals from the gastroduodenal artery to the liver. **D** Hepatogram phase of C. Small residual tumor is still present. The patient is still alive four and one-half years later.

agement of 49 patients with metastases limited primarily to the lung and/or bone. Another 26 patients with extensive metastases, especially to the liver, were treated by renal infarction to palliate pain and hemorrhage. In a third group of 25 patients without metastases, renal artery occlusion was done immediately before nephrectomy [18, 19]. Our current approach is outlined in Figure 5.

Extent of Disease

Local Tumor (No Metastases). Eight of the 25 patients with localized renal carcinoma are dead after

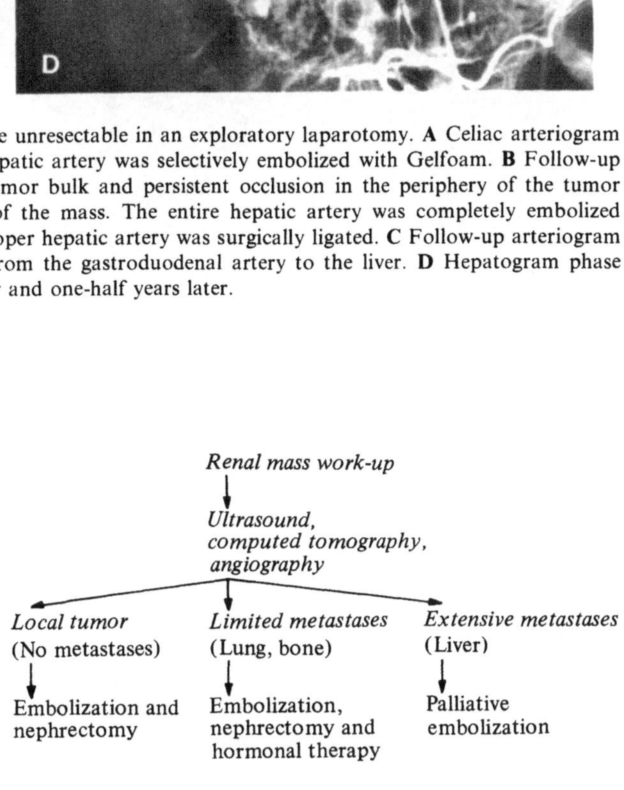

Renal mass work-up

↓

*Ultrasound,
computed tomography,
angiography*

Local tumor (No metastases)	*Limited metastases* (Lung, bone)	*Extensive metastases* (Liver)
Embolization and nephrectomy	Embolization, nephrectomy and hormonal therapy	Palliative embolization

Fig. 5. Approach in cases with renal masses.

65

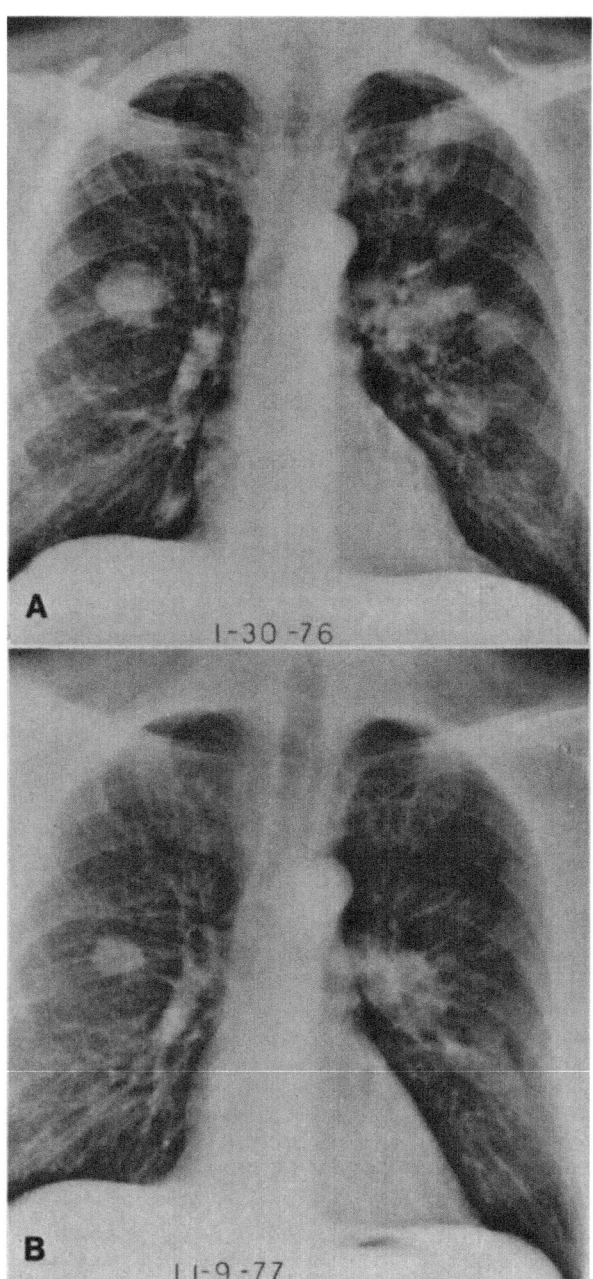

Fig. 6A and B. Renal carcinoma with pulmonary metastases. **A** Multiple metastatic nodules in both lungs. The primary renal carcinoma was infarcted and resected; subsequently, the patient was given hormonal therapy (Depo-provera). **B** Follow-up chest film 20 months later revealed a decrease in the size and number of lung metastases (partial response). The patient is still alive with residual pulmonary metastases four years later.

a median survival of 19 months. In ten living patients, the median follow-up period is 22 months. The remaining seven patients are still alive, but the follow-up period is too short for an evaluation (a minimum of four months is necessary). Since this group of pa-

tients has not yet reached the median survival curve, a conclusion cannot be drawn at present.

Limited Metastases Group. The majority of these patients had metastases to lung and bone; rare metastatic sites included skin, lymph nodes, and vena cava. This group of 49 patients was treated by renal infarction, nephrectomy, and progesterone. The infarction was done using a combination of Gelfoam and steel coils, with nephrectomy performed four to seven days later (range: 0–11 days). Postoperatively, progesterone (Depo-Provera) hormonal therapy was administered to all patients.

Complete response (CR) of the pulmonary metastases (for at least six months) occurred in 12% of patients and partial remission (greater than 50% reduction of metastases for at least six months) in 10%. Stable disease (a 25% change in the pulmonary metastases over at least one year) was observed in 14%. The total 36% response rate in this group of patients is far superior to any other results in Stage IV disease. Figure 6 illustrates a patient with partial response of his pulmonary metastasis.

Extensive Metastases Group. Metastasis to the liver (14%) is an ominous sign that has been refractory to all treatment modalities, including renal infarction. Also included in this group are patients with contralateral renal or diffuse abdominal metastases. Palliative infarction is done to control gross hematuria and/or persistent flank pain. The median survival of this group was four to five months.

Complications

Virtually all patients who undergo arterial occlusion experienced flank pain of 24–48 hours duration, requiring narcotics for relief. The narcotics are given intravenously in aliquots of 25 mg meperidine hydrochloride (Demerol) during embolization. Fever up to 40° C almost always accompanies the pain, and lasts as long as five days, but antibiotics are seldom needed. Anorexia, nausea, and vomiting may occur for three to five days, requiring symptomatic management. In a few patients, paralytic ileus may require nasogastric suction and intravenous fluids. Hypertension occurs in many patients during embolization and lasts two to four hours; no patient has experienced persistent hypertension.

Major complications have been relatively few. Renal failure occurred early in the series in two patients, in one of whom it was irreversible. This was believed to be related to the large volume of contrast material used (300 ml) and to the infarction that was performed at the same time. For the last 80 patients, the diagnostic and interventional procedures have been separated by at least 48 hours, and no other episode of failure has occurred. Renal abscess complicated occlusion in two patients, with one fatality occurring due to Gram-negative septicemia. A pre-existing pyuria was held responsible. Consequently, in the presence of a urinary tract infection, antibiotics are given one week before and after embolization. The second patient had no fever or pain, and speckled gas in the kidney was therefore attributed to tumor necrosis rather than to abscess.

Unintentional embolization of the Gelfoam and steel coils is always a potential complication. A balloon catheter has been used by some to minimize the likelihood of escape of Gelfoam particles. This measure was not employed in this series because the Gelfoam was used only to embolize the periphery of the tumor with central occlusion accomplished with a coil. Loss of a coil occurred in one patient; Chuang has developed a method for extracting the errant stainless steel coil using a Dormier basket [20].

Bone

Transcatheter management of primary and secondary bone tumors includes both arterial infusion and occlusion. Intraarterial infusion of chemotherapeutic agents has been used primarily in malignant bone tumors, and arterial occlusion has been effective in giant cell tumors and aneurysmal bone cysts. Bone pain has been controlled by arterial occlusion of metastatic renal cell carcinoma [21].

Intraarterial Infusion of Malignant Bone Tumors

Technique. Transfemoral catheterization using a 5 or 6.5 French catheter is the usual approach. Contralateral femoral puncture is frequently preferred, with antegrade catheterization over the bifurcation of the aorta to the ipsilateral pelvic and lower extremity vessels. If the bone tumor is supplied by a single feeding artery, then selective catheterization is optimal.

Infusion

CDDP is infused at a dosage of 120 mg/m² over a two to 24-hour period with the patient on vigorous hydration and mannitol diuresis. The infusion is repeated at three-to-four-week intervals for three or four courses [22]. In patients who failed to respond to the infusion or who developed drug toxicity, another therapeutic regimen was instituted – methotrexate, 7.5 to 10 g/m² with citrovorum rescue (N. Jaffe et al., unpublished data).

Results. In 14 patients with osteosarcoma, eight (57%) had a significant response to CDDP. In six of the nine patients, the response was documented by surgical and histologic examination in five and by cytologic examination of a specimen obtained by percutaneous biopsy in one (V.P. Chuang et al., unpublished data). Figure 7 illustrates a patient with partial response to CDDP. Seven other patients with a variety of malignant bone tumors, including chondrosarcoma and malignant fibrohistiocytoma were treated with CDDP with a similar response.

Complications. Two patients developed skin reactions with edema and discoloration and one patient experienced severe myelosuppression. In four patients, all children, transient hypertension was noted. Neurologic, auditory, or nephrogenic CDDP toxicity was not manifested in this series.

Comment. The historical three-year survival rate for osteosarcoma treated by immediate resection or a combination of radiation therapy and surgery is no greater than 20%. With improved chemotherapy, yielding a 50% three-year survival rate, conservative surgical resection has been incorporated into the present protocol. Preoperative control of the primary tumor by CDDP infusion is followed by a limb salvage procedure. A customized endoprosthesis is utilized to preserve limb function (V.P. Chuang, unpublished data).

Embolic Occlusion of Benign Bone Tumors

Benign bone tumors, including giant cell tumors and aneurysmal bone cysts, were treated by arterial occlusion in eleven patients. These tumors involved predominantly the innominate bone, sacrum, and distal lumbar spine.

Embolization Technique. Following a diagnostic arteriogram, arterial embolization is initiated with 3-mm cubes of Gelfoam. When the flow slows, larger Gelfoam strips (5 × 5 × 20 mm) are compressed and injected through a 1-ml syringe. With the catheter well seated in the artery, stainless steel coils are inserted to complete the arterial occlusion; a 5 French minicoil has been used in smaller vessels, e.g., the lumbar arteries. Embolization is performed only from the third lumbar vertebra and below for fear of uninten-

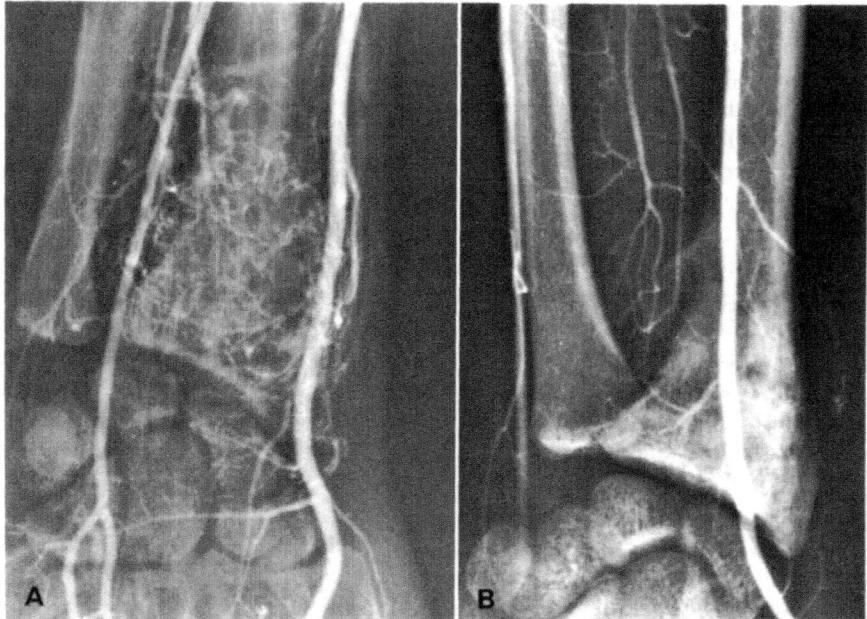

Fig. 7A and B. Osteosarcoma of left radius. **A** Left brachial arterigram shows multiple tumor vessels from the radial and ulnar arteries. Three courses of CDDP were given at monthly intervals. The pain completely subsided following the first course of treatment. **B** Follow-up arteriogram after the third course of CDDP. No tumor vessels are seen. In addition there is an overall increased density (calcification) of the tumor. Resection revealed 70% tumor necrosis (partial response).

tional occlusion of the anterior spinal artery with resultant paraplegia.

Results. Ten of the eleven patients are evaluable; six of the ten, 60%, responded to arterial occlusion. The response was manifested by pain relief, decrease in tumor size, and calcification in the rim of the tumor. One patient has remained asymptomatic for four years.

Complications. Adverse reactions occurred in three patients, with a foot drop occurring in two and transient numbness in one. Many of these patients experienced pain that was different from that experienced prior to embolization and that persisted for a few days.

Pelvic Neoplasms

Intraarterial therapy via bilateral internal iliac artery infusion has been of benefit in the treatment of tumors in the pelvis, including carcinomas of the bladder, prostate, cervix, and ovary, and recurrent colon carcinoma.

Bladder

Carcinoma of the bladder, when confined to the bladder, is treated by radiation therapy followed by cystec-

tomy in six weeks with a 50% five-year survival rate. In the presence of disease beyond the bladder, radiation therapy alone will yield a 16% five-year survival rate. In diffuse metastases or following failure of the previously described management, chemotherapy (CDDP, adriamycin, and cyclophosphamide) is administered systemically. This regime is more effective against the metastases, especially pulmonary, than against the primary transitional cell carcinoma. To palliate the pain and hemorrhage of the recurrent or residual carcinoma of the bladder, bilateral internal iliac artery infusion was attempted in 21 patients.

Technique. Each internal iliac artery is catheterized with a 5 or 6.5 French catheter, usually from the ipsilateral femoral artery. On occasion, placement is better accomplished from each contralateral femoral artery. Each catheter is connected to a separate pump to permit equivalent delivery of the chemotherapeutic agents. CDDP is infused at a rate of 80–150 mg/m^2 (usually 120 mg/m^2) over a 24-hour period, divided between the two catheters. Mannitol and hydration are also administered to prevent possible renal and neurotoxicity.

Results. Patients with recurrent disease of the bladder after failure of radiation therapy and/or surgery who were admitted to MDAH because of pain and hematuria usually survived approximately three months.

Twenty-one patients were treated by intraarterial infusion. Pain relief was accomplished in 18 of the 21. Three patients succumbed to the disease, and 17 are still alive as long as one year after the initiation of treatment. Two patients who failed to respond to CDDP, one with signet ring adenocarcinoma of the bladder and the other with transitional cell carcinoma, did respond dramatically to a combined intraarterial administration of 5-FU and intravenous infusion of mitomycin C and adriamycin.

References

1. Jaffe, G.M., Donegan, W.L., Watson, F., Spratt, G.S.: Factors influencing survival in patients with untreated hepatic metastases. Surg. Gynecol. Obstet. 127:1–11, 1968
2. Ansfield, F.J., Ramiriz, G., Skibba, J.L., Davis, H.L., Wirtanen, G.W.: Intrahepatic arterial infusion with 5-Fluorouracil. Cancer 28:1147–1151, 1971
3. Frei, E., III: Effect of dose and schedule on response. In: Cancer medicine, edited by J.F. Holland and E. Frei III. Philadelphia, Lea and Febiger, 1973
4. Healy, J.E.: Vascular patterns in human metastatic liver tumors. Surg. Gynecol. Obstet. 120:1187–1193, 1965
5. Nilsson, L.A.: Therapeutic hepatic artery ligation in patients with secondary liver tumors. Rev. Surg. 23:374–376, 1966
6. Ensminger, W.D., Rosovsky, A., Raso, V., Leven, D.C., Glode, M., Come, S., Steele, G., Frei, E., III: A clinical-pharmacological evaluation of hepatic arterial infusions of 5-Fluoro-21-Deoxyuridine and 5-Fluorouracil. Cancer Res. 38:3784–3792, 1978
7. Patt, Y.Z., Mavligit, G.M., Chuang, V.P., Wallace, S., Johnston, S., Benjamin, R.S., Valdivieso, M., Hersh, E.M.: Percutaneous hepatic arterial infusion (HAI) of Mitomycin C and Floxuridine (FUDR): An effective treatment for metastatic colorectal carcinoma of the liver. Cancer 46:29–33, 1980
8. Calvo, D.B., Patt, Y.Z., Wallace, S., Chuang, V.P., Benjamin, R.S., Pritchard, J.D., Hersh, E.M., Bodey, G.P., Mavligitt, G.M.: Phase I trial of percutaneous intra-arterial (IA) cis-diamminedichloride-platinum (II) (CDDP) for regionally confined malignancies. Cancer 45:1278–1283, 1980
9. Chuang, V.P., Wallace, S.: Hepatic arterial redistribution for intraarterial infusion of hepatic neoplasm. Radiology 135:295–299, 1980
10. Michels, N.A.: Blood supply and anatomy of the upper abdominal organs. Philadelphia, Lippincott, 1955
11. Anderson, J.H., Wallace, S., Gianturco, C., Gerson, L.P.: "Mini" Gianturco stainless steel coils for transcatheter vascular occlusion. Radiology 132:301–303, 1979
12. Chuang, V.P., Wallace, S., Gianturco, C.: A new improved coil for tapered-tip catheter for arterial occlusion. Radiology 135:507–509, 1980
13. Lee, Y.T.N.: Nonsystemic treatment of metastatic tumors of the liver – a review. Med. Pediat. Oncol. 4:185–203, 1978
14. Mori, W., Masuda, M., Miyanaga, T.: Hepatic artery ligation and tumor necrosis in the liver. Surgery 59:359–363, 1966
15. Hrushesky, W.J., Murphy, G.P.: Current status of the therapy of advanced renal carcinoma. J. Surg. Oncol. 9:277–288, 1977
16. Johnson, D.E., Samuels, M.L.: Chemotherapy for metastatic renal carcinoma. In: Cancer Chemotherapy: Fundamental concepts and recent advances (Proceedings of The University of Texas System Cancer Center, M.D. Anderson Hospital and Tumor Institute 19th Annual Clinical Conference on Cancer, 1975), Chicago, Year Book Medical Publishers, Inc. 1975, pp. 493–503
17. Johnson, D.E., Kaesler, K.E., Samuels, M.L.: Is nephrectomy justified in patients with metastatic renal carcinoma? J. Urol. 114:27–29, 1975
18. Wallace, S., Chuang, V.P., Bracken, B., Hersh, E.M., Ayala, A., Johnson, D.: Embolization of renal carcinoma: Experience with 100 patients. Radiology (in press, 1980)
19. Wallace, S., Chuang, V.P., Green, B., Swanson, D.A., Bracken, R.B., Johnson, D.E.: Diagnostic radiology in renal carcinoma. In: Cancer of the Genitourinary Tract, edited by D.E. Johnson and M.L. Samuels. New York, Raven Press, 1979, p. 33–45
20. Chuang, V.P.: Nonoperative retrieval of Gianturco coils from abdominal aorta. Am. J. Roentgenol. 132:996–997, 1979
21. Chuang, V.P., Wallace, S., Swanson, D., Zornoza, J., Handel, F.H., Schwarten, D.A., Murray, J.: Arterial occlusion in the management of pain from metastatic renal carcinoma. Radiology 133:611–614, 1979
22. Chuang, V.P., Wallace, S., Benjamin, R.S., Jaffe, N.: Therapeutic intraarterial infusion of Cis-platinum in the management of malignant bone tumors: A preliminary report (abstract). Presented at the 27th Annual Meeting of the Association of University Radiologists, Rochester, NY, 1979

Comment

Current Status of Transcatheter Management of Neoplasms: A Surgeon's View

Alfred M. Cohen

Department of Surgery, Harvard Medical School and Surgical Services, Massachusetts General Hospital, Boston, Massachusetts, USA

Drs. Chuang and Wallace present an overview of an increasingly complex multidisciplinary area that is of interest to medical and surgical oncologists and radiation therapists as well as to radiologists. Interventional angiographic techniques often allow complex, aggressive treatment programs to be carried out in ill patients with limited life expectancies without subjecting these patients to major surgery. I will limit my further comments to the area of the liver malignancies.

The authors describe various approaches to the treatment of hepatic neoplasms by arterial occlusions. Central arterial occlusion using a spring device or glue injection, or more peripheral occlusion using Gelfoam embolization may be complementary. Whether such transcatheter techniques are as effective as surgical devascularization of the liver remains unclear. There is little doubt, however, that arterial occlusion can result in tumor necrosis and may be particularly valuable in treatment of patients with hormone-producing metastases, such as carcinoids. It is also intriguing to speculate on the role of hepatic artery thrombosis or peripheral embolization during arterial infusion chemotherapy. In patients who have had long-term infusion chemotherapy via hepatic artery catheters serial angiograms document a high incidence of thrombosis. Future studies involving regional chemotherapy should investigate the arterial status in all patients who have allegedly responded to the infusion chemotherapy.

Infusion chemotherapy of liver tumors has usually involved long-term hepatic artery drug infusions. Some surgical oncology groups have been interested in hepatic artery ligation and portal vein infusion, which is an area yet to be explored by radiologists.

Certainly arterial occlusion and transhepatic portal vein catheterization can be performed angiographically.

The steep dose-response curve for the fluoropyrimidines and the high extraction ratio of the liver makes fluorodeoxyuridine an ideal drug for arterial treatment. Hepatic artery–to–peripheral vein concentration ratios of over 40 to 1 can be obtained in the steady state situation. The use of prolonged, continuous infusions, however, is not appropriate for all drugs. The nitrosoureas' effectiveness is related to peak concentration. Other drugs with long half-lives and minimal hepatic extraction, such as methotrexate, also provide little benefit when given by hepatic arterial infusion. Clearly, in the future, clinical pharmacologists and medical oncologists must work closely with radiologists in devising more suitable treatment programs.

An additional variable in arterial infusion chemotherapy is the use of anticoagulants. The use of anticoagulants to prevent experimental metastases is well established, but it is not widely known that some of these agents, such as warfarin (Coumadin) directly inhibit tumor growth. The M.D. Anderson group uses significant amounts of heparin in their patients, and the effects of this drug on primary tumor growth is unknown.

Another aspect of considerable practical importance that was not commented upon by the authors is the distribution of drug to the liver during hepatic artery chemotherapy. The angiography catheter is usually positioned just distal to the take-off of the gastroduodenal artery, which may place it in close proximity to the bifurcation of the left and right hepatic arteries. Streaming may produce maldistribution of the infused drug. Pressure or even hand injections of contrast dye in the angiography suite is not a reliable indicator of drug distribution. A very slow injection of 2 mCi of technetium-99m labeled macroaggre-

Address reprint requests to: A.M. Cohen, M.D., Department of Sugery, Massachusetts General Hospital, Fruit Street, Boston, MA 02114, USA

gated albumin through an angiography catheter allows more a physiologic determination of flow distribution by liver scan technique.

The authors did not discuss the important collaboration of radiation therapists in such interventional angiographic approaches. Several groups are combining external beam radiation therapy in association with hepatic artery chemotherapy, but it is unclear whether this is better than arterial chemotherapy alone. Transcatheter injection of the beta emitter yttrium-90 microspheres as a source of internal radiation therapy continues to be explored in a few centers. The direct hepatic arterial infusion of the radiosensitizer bromodeoxyuridine has also yet to be evaluated.

The heterogeneous nature of the patients presents great difficulty in comparing series. While median survival is often compared, the percentage of patients alive two years after the beginning of treatment might provide a more significant point of comparison. If such approaches can produce an increase in the "tail" of the survival curve, we will have made real progress. At all times concerns over the comfort and convenience of the patient must be evaluated and balanced against any potential benefits. The recent availability of an entirely implantable, refillable drug infusion pump provides marked improvement in the quality of life for such patients. We have recently integrated this pump with transbrachial hepatic artery catheterization. Concomitant with further pharmacologic studies of combinations of drugs for long-term regional hepatic chemotherapy should come use of better catheter materials to minimize thrombotic and embolic complications.

The Treatment of Hyperparathyroidism by Transcatheter Techniques

John L. Doppman

Department of Diagnostic Radiology, The Clinical Center, National Institutes of Health, Bethesda, Maryland, USA

Abstract. Gelfoam embolization of parathyroid adenomas causes temporary remission of hypercalcemia, but collateral circulation revascularizes the gland. Embolization with silicone permanently infarcts the gland, but is associated with all the risks of capillary bed occlusion. The staining of parathyroid adenomas with contrast material avoids the risks of particulate embolization and appears to produce permanent ablation. We carried out embolization or staining procedures in 14 parathyroid adenomas. In three of the four cases in which Gelfoam embolization was performed, hypercalcemia recurred within six months to two years; in the fourth case, in which persistent normocalcemia has been found, intense staining had been demonstrated before embolization. In eight of the remaining 10 cases, adequate staining was achieved, and normocalcemia has been maintained in all up to 36 months.

Key words: Gelfoam – Embolism, therapeutic – Adenoma – Parathyroid, neoplasms – Catheters and catheterization – Interventional radiology.

Parathyroid adenomas are ideal targets for transcatheter therapy. Small hypervascular tumors with profound metabolic activity, they are generally supplied by a single feeding artery and are therefore unusually susceptible to ischemic injury. When their blood supply arises from an expendable artery, such as the internal mammary [1], and when their removal from the anterior mediastinum would require a sternal-splitting incision, transcatheter embolic therapy seems a reasonable alternative.

Our early experience with Gelfoam and silicone embolization was encouraging [2]. However, we felt

Address reprints requests to: J.L. Doppman, M.D., Diagnostic Radiology Department NIH, The Clinical Center, Bldg. 10, Rm. 6S211, Bethesda, MD 20205, USA

obliged to restrict embolization to anterior mediastinal adenomas with an internal mammary blood supply because of the risks of using particulate material in the thyrocervical trunk. The development of techniques to ablate glandular function by staining with an iodinated water-soluble contrast agent [3] has extended the application of transcatheter therapy, not only as an alternative to a second operation but even as a primary therapeutic option in patients who are poor surgical risks.

Methods and Results

Embolization

Simply obstructing the feeding artery to a hyperfunctioning parathyroid gland with Gelfoam does not per-

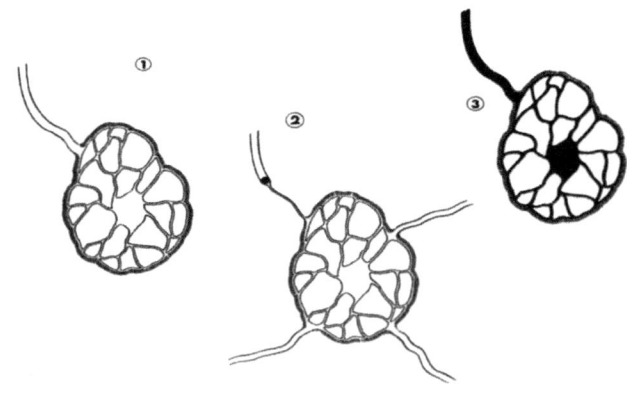

Fig. 1. Parathyroid glands have single feeding arteries entering at the hilum (1). Embolic obstruction of the solitary feeding artery (2) stimulates the development of a collateral circulation, and hyperparathyroidism generally recurs. Vascular "casting" with silicone (3) eliminates potential collaterals and permanently infarcts the gland.

manently control hypersecretion. The temporary control that may be achieved is similar to remissions in hypercalcemia that occasionally follow surgery in which no parathyroid tissue was removed. Such remissions are probably due to the inadvertent ligation of the arterial supply to the adenoma, and they are almost never permanent since a collateral circulation later develops to revascularize the gland. Permanent embolic ablation requires an agent that obturates the gland's capillary bed and excludes revascularization [4] (Fig. 1).

Our initial experience with Gelfoam embolization was encouraging (Fig. 2), but in three of the four cases in which it was performed (Cases 1, 3, and 4, Table 1), hypercalcemia recurred within six months to two years. In the single case in which Gelfoam caused permanent remission (Case 2), intense and persistent staining had been demonstrated before embolization (Fig. 3). In retrospect, the staining was considered as probably having been responsible for the auspicious result. One patient whose gland was embolized with silicone (Fig. 4) when hypercalcemia recurred six months after Gelfoam embolization remains normocalcemic three and one-half years post-silicone embolization (Case 4). Although silicone embolization is an effective technique, the use of injectable plastics in the vicinity of proximal subclavian branches exposes cerebral and spinal vascular beds to the risk of permanent occlusion.

Staining

When an artery is obstructed with a wedged or balloon catheter, very high pressures are transmitted during injection to the downstream vascular bed, and the capillaries are maximally dilated. The early, dense venous filling is often misinterpreted as evidence of arteriovenous shunts but merely reflects the shortened transit time through a maximally dilated capillary bed. Under these circumstances, extravasation of the contrast agent into the interstitial tissue occurs at an accelerated rate, and dense staining results. Both the hyperosmolarity and the chemotoxicity of essentially undiluted contrast agent produce severe and usually irreversible cellular damage (unpublished data). Since the vascular bed of even large parathyroid glands has a capacity of only a few milliliters, the manual injection of 20–30 ml of contrast agent is sufficient to stain the adenoma. Patients experience a burning sensation at the time of staining, but this quickly disappears at the conclusion of the infusion [3]. The addition of a local anesthetic agent to the perfusate, as is current practice in peripheral arteriography, may be helpful; however, significant prolonged

pain, as occurs following muscle [5] or adrenal staining, has not been a problem with parathyroid staining. Gross staining often persists up to 24 hours; more sensitive modalities, such as computed tomography [6] can detect staining for as long as 96 hours (Fig. 5). Since all capillary beds downstream from the wedged catheter are stained, and since it is sometimes not possible to isolate the adenoma's blood supply, staining of thymus and chest wall muscles will sometimes occur; this is a painful but not a serious complication [5]

Unlike embolization, staining leaves the feeding artery and vascular bed of the adenoma intact. Arteriography can be performed at a later date to evaluate the results or to repeat the staining.

Our initial experience with parathyroid staining [3] was confined to adenomas in the anterior mediastinum whose removal would have required splitting the sternum (Fig. 6). The arterial supply arose from the thymic branch of the internal mammary artery. Wedging was easily achieved, and was, in fact, usually unavoidable, with a 5 French catheter. When separate thymic and thyroid isthmic branches arose proximally, the artery to the adenoma had to be selectively catheterized for successful staining (Fig. 7).

Intense staining can usually be achieved by the manual injection over 20–30 seconds of 30 ml of sodium and meglumine diatrizoate (Renografin-76). If minor reflux into the internal mammary artery occurs, staining can still be achieved by increasing the volume and rate of infusion. If free reflux occurs, staining cannot be accomplished without recourse to a double-lumen balloon catheter. This was never required in our experience.

It is feasible to stain adenomas in the neck, provided the feeding artery can be selectively catheterized. Glands in the posterior-superior mediastinum often derive their arterial supply from the caudal loop of the thyrocervical trunk. Figure 8 illustrates staining of a left cervical parathyroid adenoma in a patient (Case 12) whose left thyroid lobe had been resected at the initial unsuccessful cervical exploration.

In a single instance (Case 13), retrograde venous staining [7] of an anterior mediastinal adenoma was performed when selective arterial catheterization could not be achieved. A rather dramatic outpouring of parathyroid hormone (PTH) was documented immediately after venous staining, but this probably also occurs following arterial staining (Fig. 9). Quantities of PTH stored in parathyroid adenomas are not sufficient to precipitate acute hypercalcemia even with total discharge. We have documented short-lived PTH elevations following arterial staining and embolization, but acute hypercalcemia has never occurred. In this patient hypercalcemia recurred three months

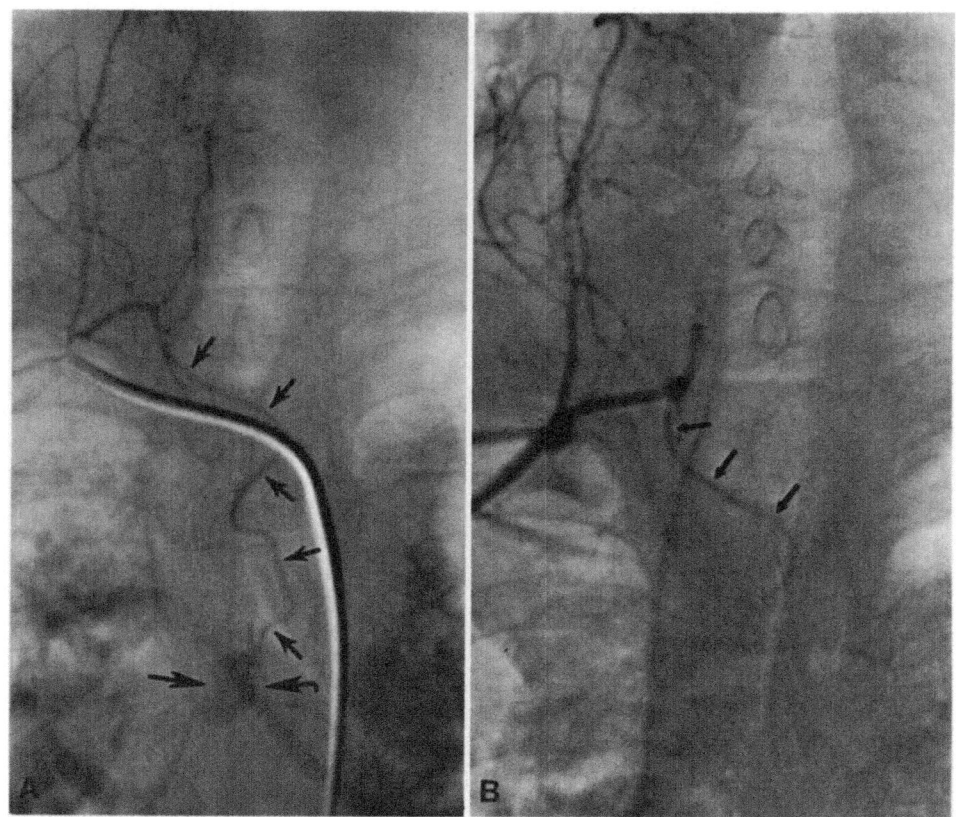

Fig. 2A and B. A Descending thymic branch (*small arrows*) of the right inferior thyroid artery is shown supplying a small anterior mediastinal adenoma (*large arrows*). The right thyroid lobe had been removed at an initial unsuccessful operation. **B** The feeding artery (*arrows*) is shown after embolization from an axillary approach with Gelfoam. The catheter was never wedged; thus, parathyroid staining is absent. The patient remained normocalcemic for one year but then hypercalcemia recurred.

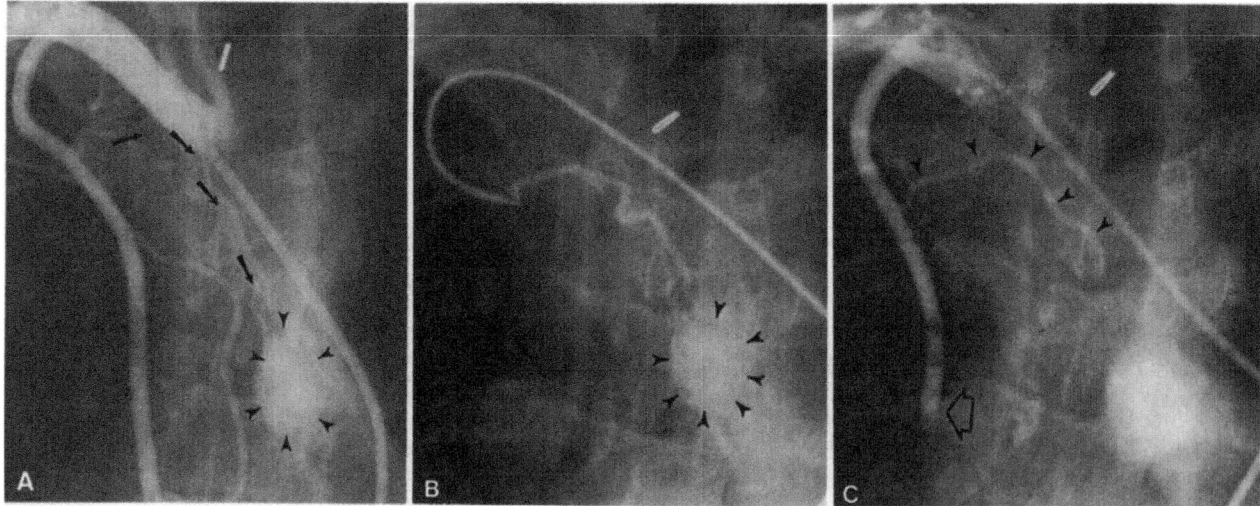

Fig. 3A–C. Case 2. **A** An anterior mediastinal adenoma (*arrowheads*) is shown supplied by the thymic branch of the right internal mammary artery (*arrows*). **B** After selective catheterization of the artery, the gland was inadvertently stained (*arrowheads*). **C** The feeding artery (*arrowheads*) has been embolized with Gelfoam. Note the incidental embolic occlusion of the internal mammary artery (*open arrowhead*); reflux of particulate agents is difficult to avoid when embolizing small vessels. The patient remains normocalcemic five years after embolization.

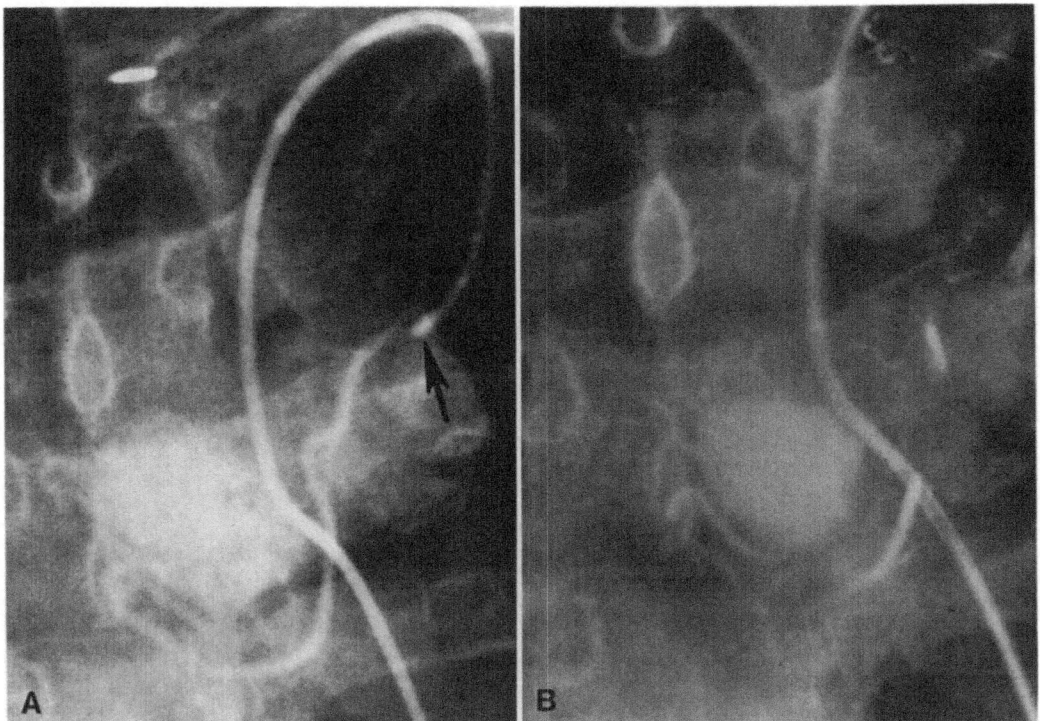

Fig. 4A and B. Case 4. **A** Selective arteriogram of an anterior mediastinal adenoma (*arrow*). Gelfoam embolization was performed, but hyperparathyroidism recurred six months later. **B** In a second procedure, the were adenoma and feeding artery were filled with opaque silicone rubber; normocalcemia has persisted for three and one-half years.

Table 1. Results of embolization or staining procedures in 14 patients with hyperparathyroidism

Case	Sex	Age	Date of Intervention	Site of adenoma	Arterial supply	Embolization	Staining	Current status
1	F	36	Oct. '73	Anterior mediastinum	Inferior thyroid	Gelfoam	0	Hypercalcemia recurred 12 months
2	F	36	Aug. '74	Anterior mediastinum	Internal mammary	Gelfoam	2 +	Normocalcemic
3	M	30	June '75	Anterior mediastinum	Internal mammary	Gelfoam	0	Hypercalcemia recurred 14 months
4	M	50	April '76	Anterior mediastinum	Internal mammary	Gelfoam followed by silicone	0	Normocalcemic
5	M	57	April '77	Anterior mediastinum	Internal mammary	0	1 +	Hypercalcemia recurred 3 months
6	F	37	Sept. '77	Anterior mediastinum	Internal mammary	0	1 +	Hypercalcemia recurred 4 months
7	M	41	April '77	Anterior mediastinum	Internal mammary	0	3 +	Normocalcemic
8	F	79	Nov. '77	Anterior mediastinum	Internal mammary	0	2 +	Normocalcemic
9	M	63	Jan. '78	Anterior mediastinum	Internal mammary	0	3 +	Normocalcemic
10	F	33	May '78	Anterior mediastinum	Internal mammary	0	3 +	Normocalcemic
11	F	56	Sept. '78	Anterior mediastinum	Internal mammary	0	4 +	Normocalcemic
12	F	46	Sept. '78	Cervical	Inferior thyroid	0	2 +	Normocalcemic
13	F	59	Dec. '78	Anterior mediastinum	Never demonstrated	0	2 + (venous)	Hypercalcemia recurred 3 months
14	F	54	May '79	Anterior mediastinum	Internal mammary	0	2 +	Normocalcemic

after venous staining. Permanent ablation probably cannot be achieved from the venous side.

Nine mediastinal (Cases 2,5–11 and 14) and one cervical (Case 12) parathyroid gland have been stained to date from the arterial side. The first two (Cases 5 and 6) occurred serendipitously, and hypercalcemia recurred within three to six months. In eight cases with adequate staining (2+ or higher, Table 1)

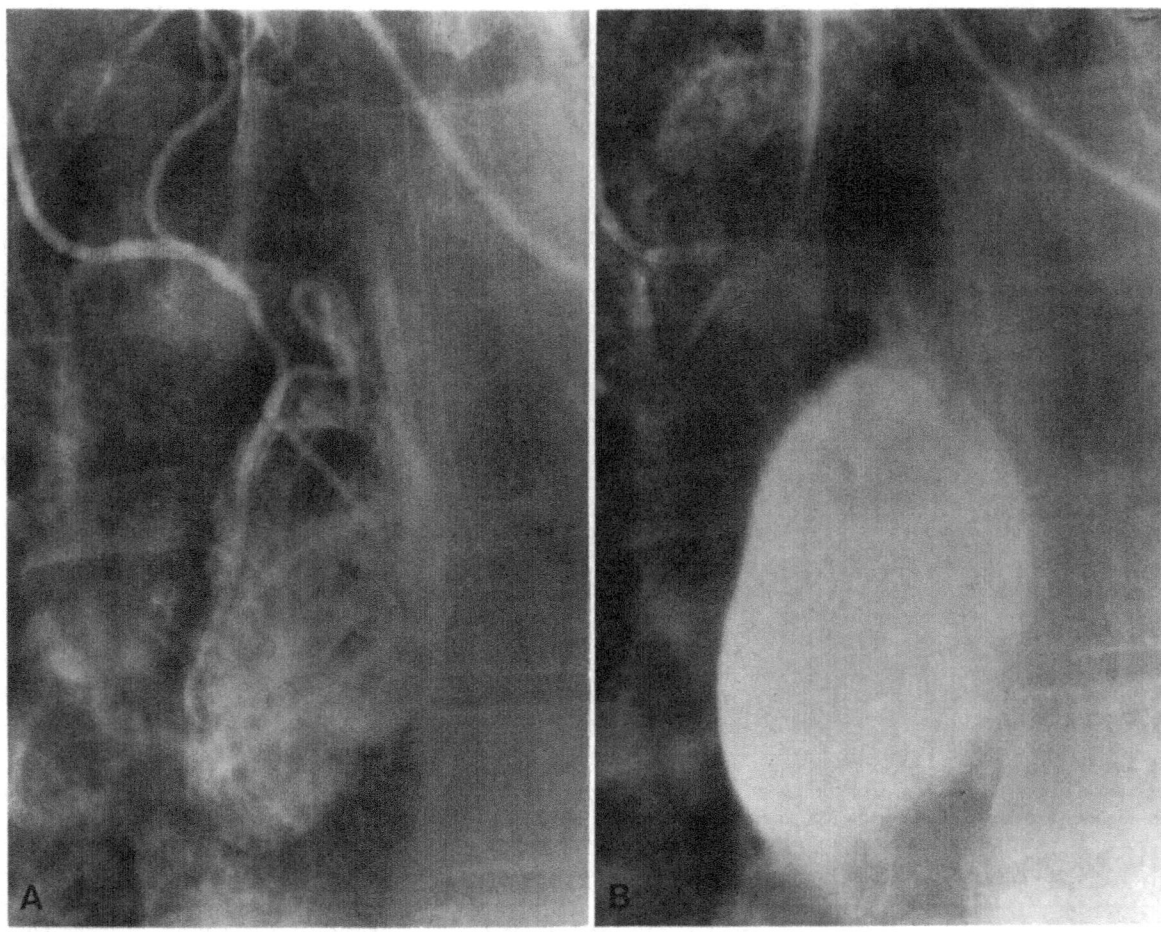

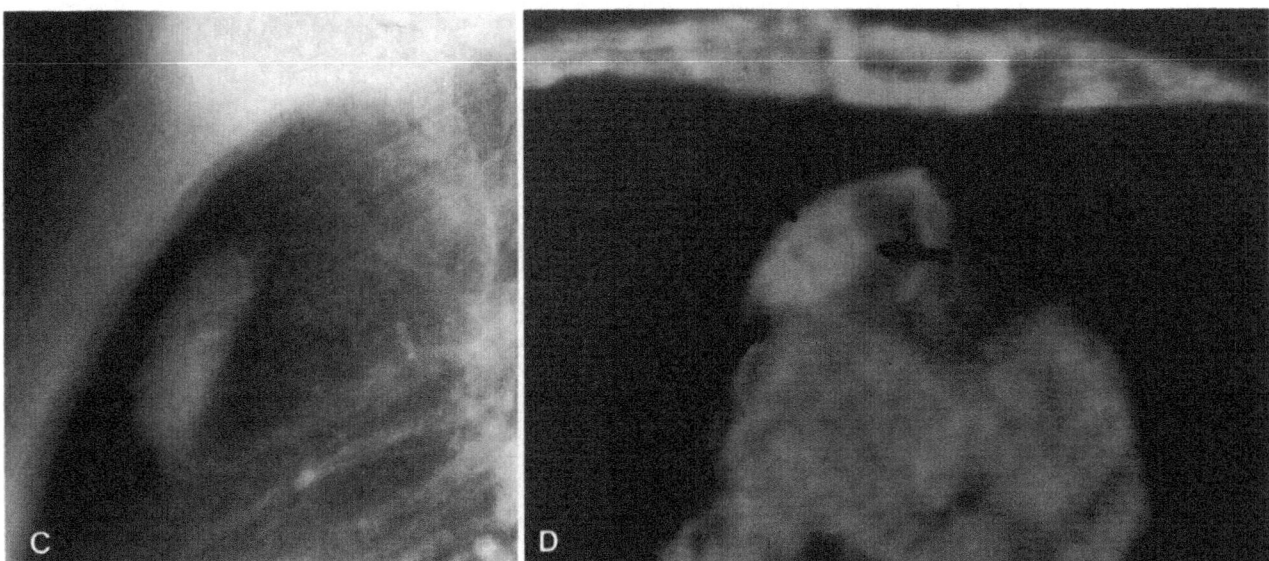

Fig. 5A–D. A A large anterior mediastinal adenoma is shown supplied by the thymic branch of the right internal mammary artery. **B** Dense opacification of the adenoma is demonstrated 15 minutes after staining. **C** Twenty-four hours later, the adenoma remains intensely stained. **D** Computed tomography, performed 96 hours later, reveals the adenoma (*arrows*) as still densely stained.

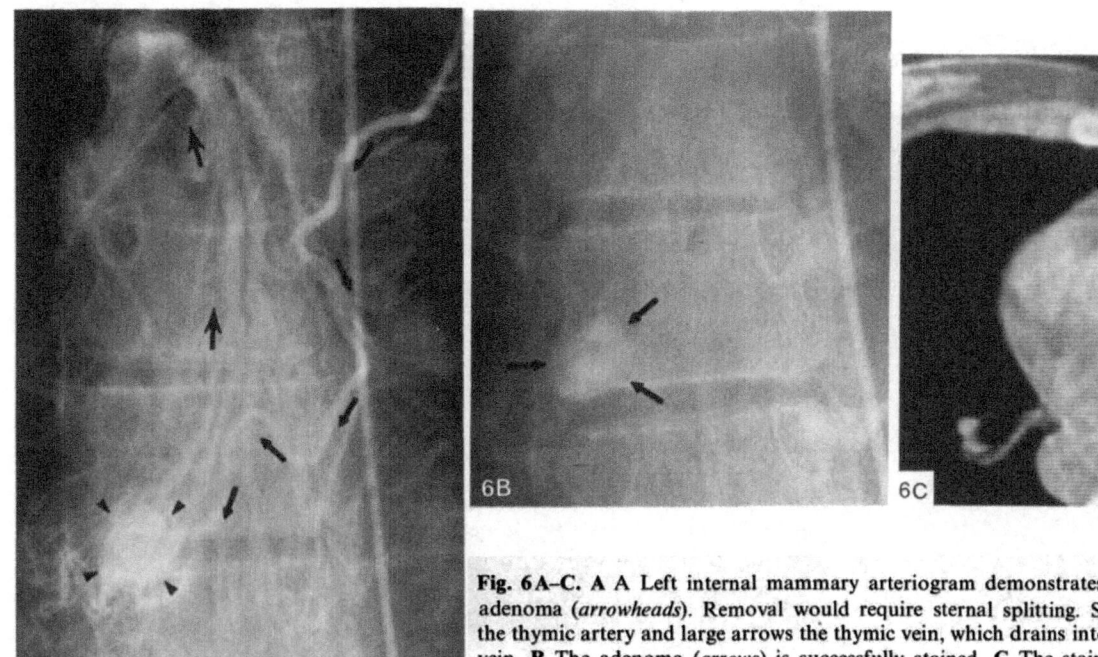

Fig. 6A–C. A A Left internal mammary arteriogram demonstrates a deep mediastinal adenoma (*arrowheads*). Removal would require sternal splitting. Small arrows identify the thymic artery and large arrows the thymic vein, which drains into the left innominate vein. **B** The adenoma (*arrows*) is successfully stained. **C** The stain (*arrow*) persists on computed tomography 24 hours later. The patient remains normocalcemic two years later.

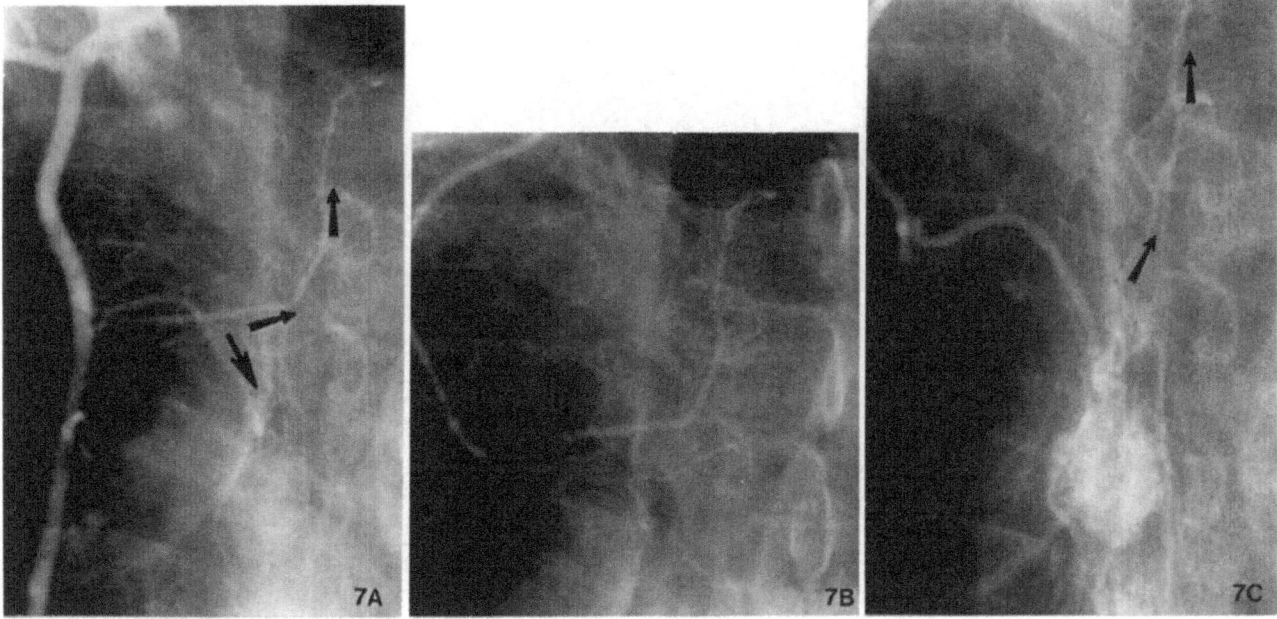

Fig. 7A–C. A Separate origins of the thymic (*large arrows*) and thyroid isthmic branches (*small arrows*) are demonstrated. **B** Wedge arteriography of the branch to the thyroid isthmus fails to stain the adenoma. **C** Successful wedge arteriography of the thymic branch stains the adenoma. Arrows identify draining thymic vein.

normocalcemia has been maintained up to 36 months. Relapse has not occurred in this deliberately stained arterial group, but longer follow-up periods are needed.

We have restricted this technique to patients with known adenomas (normal or atrophic parathyroid glands removed at previous operations) or a solitary remaining hyperplastic gland. This technique probably has no place in the treatment of multiglandular hyperplasia.

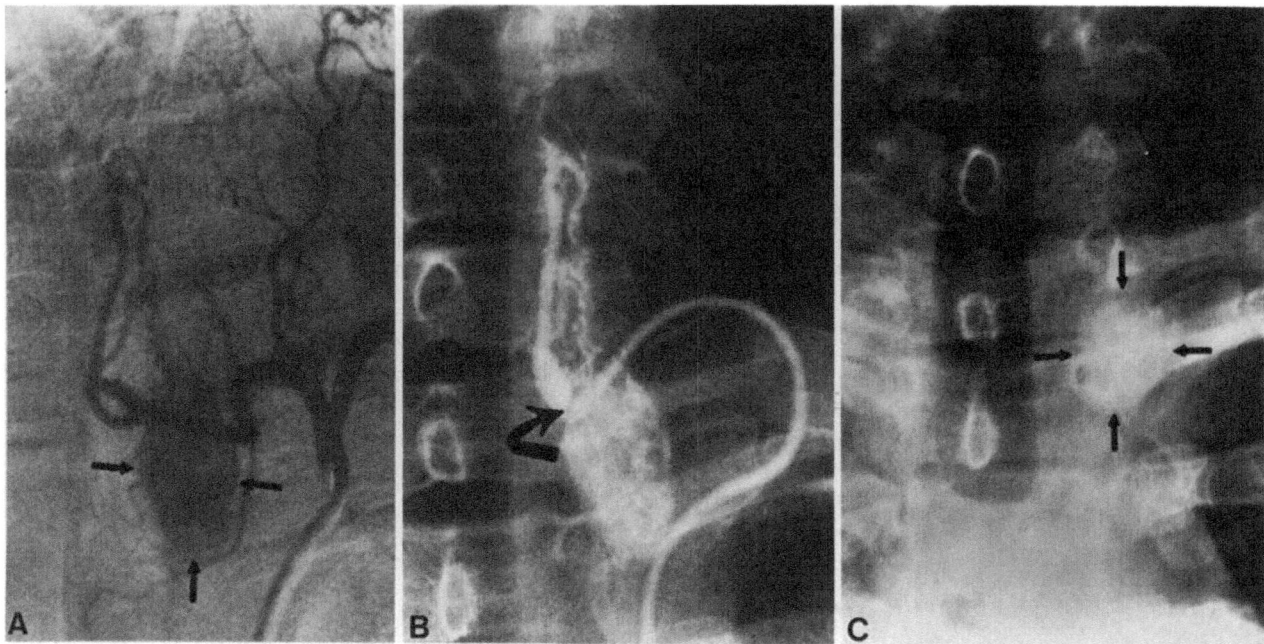

Fig. 8A–C. A An adenoma of the left posterior superior mediastinum (*arrows*) is shown supplied by the inferior thyroid artery. Left thyroid lobectomy had been performed at a previous unsuccessful operation. **B** The catheter is advanced deeply and successfully wedged (*curved arrow*) to stain the adenoma. **C** The stain (*arrows*) persists one hour later.

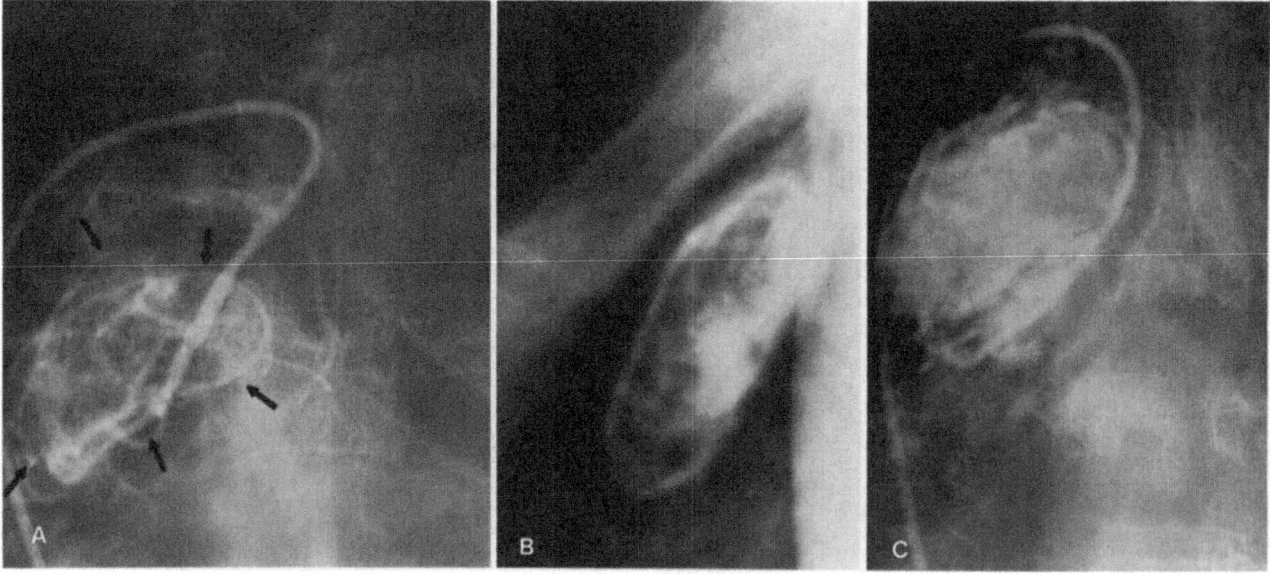

Fig. 9A–C. A A retrograde venogram demonstrates a large anterior mediastinal adenoma (*arrows*). The concentration of parathyroid hormone in the catheterized vein was high as compared to backbround levels (20.5 ng vs. 0.8 ng). **B** A lateral venogram reveals the discrete outline of the adenoma immediately behind sternum. **C** After staining there was an outpouring of parathyroid hormone from the adenoma (45.1 ng; background = 0.8 ng). Normocalcemia persisted only three months.

Risks and Complications

When all normal parathyroid glands have been removed at previous unsuccessful operations, a distressingly common phenomenon in our experience [8], staining of an adenoma results in permanent hypoparathyroidism. But so does surgical resection. Although surgery provides tissue for auto-transplantation, transplants of adenomatous tissue can cause recurrent hyperparathyroidism [9]. Since staining provides no tissue for histologic examination, the possi-

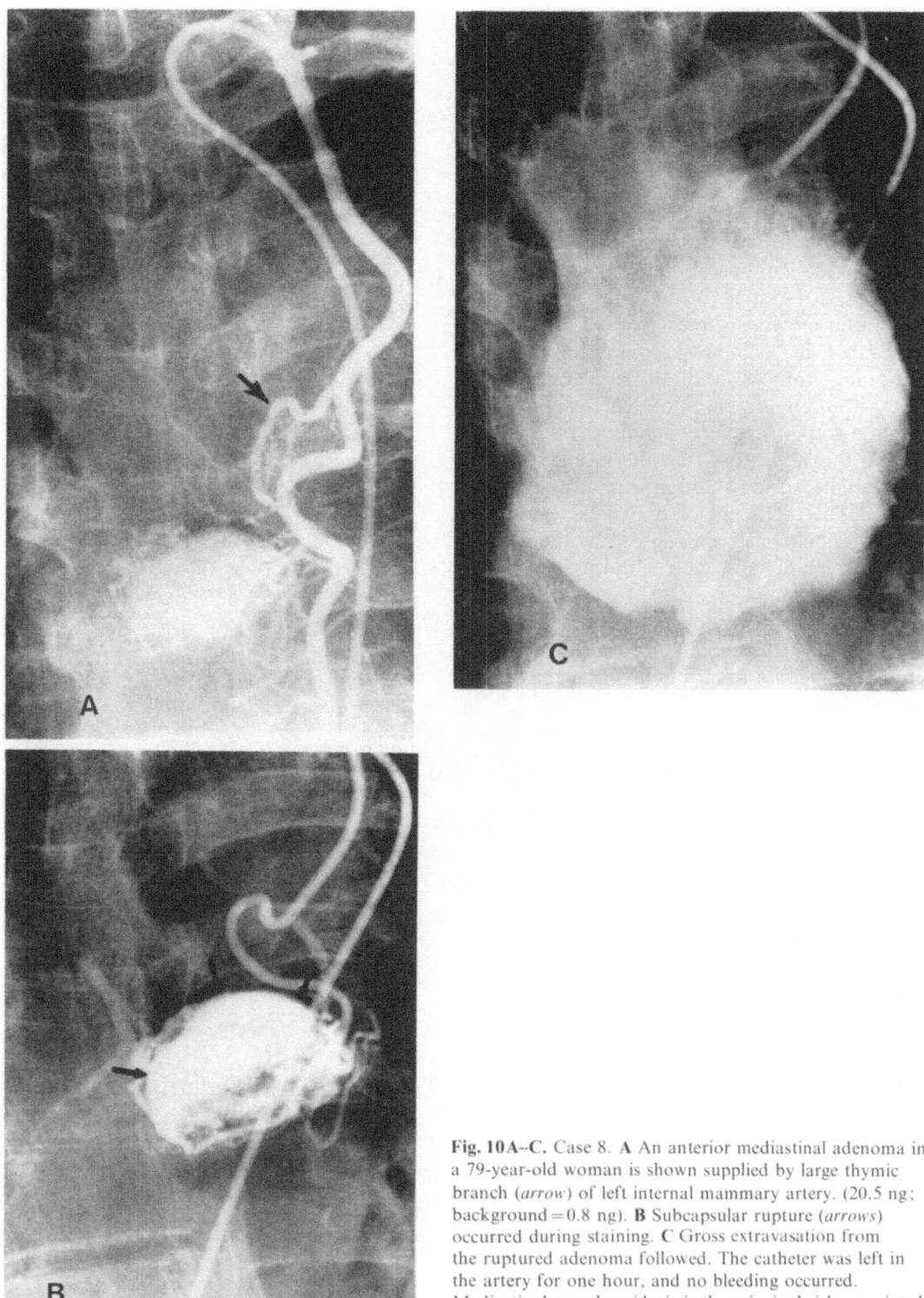

Fig. 10A–C. Case 8. **A** An anterior mediastinal adenoma in a 79-year-old woman is shown supplied by large thymic branch (*arrow*) of left internal mammary artery. (20.5 ng; background = 0.8 ng). **B** Subcapsular rupture (*arrows*) occurred during staining. **C** Gross extravasation from the ruptured adenoma followed. The catheter was left in the artery for one hour, and no bleeding occurred. Mediastinal parathyroidosis is the principal risk associated with rupture.

bility of staining a parathyroid carcinoma exists. Statistically, however, this is a very remote possibility.

Capsular rupture during staining occurred in a 79-year-old woman (Case 8) when the perfusion was not fluoroscopically monitored (Fig. 10). This is an avoidable complication. Bleeding following rupture can be easily controlled with the in situ catheter, but implantation of parathyroid cells throughout the mediastinum is a very real risk following rupture. However, this patient remains normocalcemic 24 months after the episode.

Comments

Our clinical experience with staining has been limited to the treatment of parathyroid adenomas in patients with previous unsuccessful operations. We would not hesitate, however, to stain a mediastinal adenoma in a patient without previous surgery, if such a lesion were demonstrated by computed tomography [6]. Other functioning tumors without arteriovenous shunting, e.g., islet cell or carcinoid metastases in the liver, might also be treated by staining. We have demonstrated in the laboratory that the kidneys and spleen may be ablated using staining techniques (unpublished data). The treatment of hypersplenism by embolization techniques has been plagued by the high incidence of post-embolic abscesses, although Spigos et al. [10], and Lunderquist et al. [11] have reported some success with repeated subtotal embolizations. Splenic abscesses have not been a complication of splenic staining in the laboratory, but no clinical experience is yet available.

Acknowledgements. Many associates have contributed to these studies. I am particularly grateful to Murray Brennan, M.D., Adrian Krudy, M.D., Steven Marx, M.D., Allen Spiegel, M.D., and Gerry Aurbach, M.D. for their continuous support and collaboration.

References

1. Doppman, J.L., Marx, S.J., Brennan, M., Beazley, R.M., Geelhoed, G., Aurbach, G.D.: The blood supply of mediastinal parathyroid adenomas. Ann. Surg. 185:488–490, 1977
2. Doppman, J.L., Marx, S.J., Spiegel, A.M., Mallette, L.E., Wolfe, B.A., Aurbach, G.D.: Treatment of hyperparathyroidism by percutaneous embolization of a mediastinal adenoma. Radiology 115:37–42, 1975
3. Doppman, J.L., Brown, E.M., Brennan, M.F., Spiegel, A., Marx, S.J., Aurbach, G.D.: Angiographic ablation of parathyroid adenomas. Radiology 130:577–582, 1979
4. Doppman, J.L., Zapol, W., Pierce, J.: Transcatheter embolization with a silicone rubber preparation: Experimental observations. Invest. Radiol. 6:304–309, 1971
5. Doppman, J.L., Di Chiro, G.: Paraspinal muscle infarction: A painful complication of lumbar artery embolization associated with pathognomic radiographic and laboratory findings. Radiology 119:609–613, 1976
6. Doppman, J.L., Brennan, M.F., Koehler, J.L., Marx, S.J.: CT scanning for parathyroid localization. J. Comput. Assist. Tomogr. 1:30–36, 1977
7. Shimkin, P.M., Doppman, J.L., Powell, D., Marx, S.J., Ketcham, A.S.: Demonstration of parathyroid adenomas by retrograde thyroid venography. Radiology 103:63–67, 1972
8. Doppman, J.L.: Parathyroid localization arteriography and venous sampling. Radiol. Clin. North Am. 14:163–188, 1976
9. Brennan, M.F., Brown, E.M., Marx, S.J., Spiegel, A.M., Broadus, A.E., Doppman, J.L., Weber, B., Aurbach, G.D.: Recurrent hyperparathyroidism from an autotransplanted parathyroid adenoma. N. Engl. J. Med. 299:1057–1059, 1978
10. Spigos, D.G., Jonasson, O., Mozes, M., Capek, V.: Partial splenic embolization in the treatment of hypersplenism. Am. J. Roentgenol. 132:777–782, 1979
11. Lunderquist, A.: Splenic embolization. Presented at 4th Annual Meeting of Society of Cardiovascular Radiology, Dorado Beach, Puerto Rico, 1979

Comment

The Treatment of Hyperparathyroidism by Transcatheter Techniques: A Surgeon's View

Chiu-an Wang

Department of Surgery, Harvard Medical School, and Surgical Services, Massachusetts General Hospital, Boston, Massachusetts, USA

Transcatheter embolization with Gelfoam or silicone has been used in some centers as an alternative therapy in the management of patients with hyperparathy-

Address reprint requests to: C. Wang, M.D., Surgical Services, Massachusetts General Hospital, Fruit Street, Boston, MA 02114, USA

roidism. These techniques when first reported were regarded as a therapeutic bonanza and, to some, surgery no longer seemed to be the only treatment for hyperparathyroidism. It was soon realized, however, that these techniques had failed to come up to expectations. Normocalcemia was achieved but, in the majority of patients, only temporarily, and the recurrence rate was high even in experienced hands. In the paper published here, Doppman reports a 75% recurrence of hypercalcemia (three of four patients) six months to two years after Gelfoam embolization and notes that the general use of silicone has been ruled out because of its high risk.

The reason for the failure of these therapeutic modalities is obvious. Their use was based on the assumption that most diseased parathyroid glands are supplied by a single feeding artery and that blockage of the blood flow to the gland would result in ischemia, infarction, necrosis, and ultimately the cure of the hyperparathyroidism. The validity of this assumption remains open to question because the parathyroid glands, whether diseased or normal, are often fed by several arteries. The diseased glands, particularly those in the dorsum of the upper pole of the thyroid, are fed by as many as three or four arteries stemming directly from the thyroid gland. Those at the posterior thyrocricoid junction and within the thymus are also supplied by many branches; together they form a vascular pedicle [1]. It is apparent that the effect from the blockage of a single artery would be minimal. Even if all the arterial branches were occluded, the result would still be temporary because a collateral circulation will ultimately develop causing revascularization of the parathyroid gland. To achieve success with these transcatheter approaches, *all* the arteries must be occluded. Technically, this is not an easy task. Small wonder that embolization with either Gelfoam or silicone has not withstood the test of time and that the long-term results have been disappointing.

In the other transcatheter approach reported in this paper, the staining technique, the overall success rate of 80% was attributed by Dr. Doppman to irreversible cellular damage caused by forcing 30 ml of undiluted sodium and meglumine diatrizoate (Renografin-76) into the parathyroid gland with the catheter in a wedged position. However, no histologic evidence is offered. It is well known that hemorrhage in adrenal glands occurs after vigorous and forceful angiographic studies with this agent, but cellular alteration in the resected specimens have been minimal. It appears likely that the effect is not due to the hypertonicity or toxicity of the agent alone but rather to ischemia resulting from arterial occlusion by the wedged catheter. If this is so, the effect of the staining therapy would almost never be permanent, and the recurrence rate would be as high as it is with the embolization technique. It would be interesting to see Dr. Doppman's results over a period longer than 36 months.

Unfortunately, none of the modalities of transcatheter therapy mentioned here provide tissue diagnosis. Without histologic confirmation of the diagnosis, one cannot be confident that the parathyroid lesion is not a rare malignancy instead of the more common adenoma. If it were a malignancy, the outcome would be disastrous. Should the forceful injection of the agent cause the capsule of the cancer to rupture, local implantation of the malignant cells would invariably ensue [2], greatly compromising the prognosis.

Since the parathyroid tumor in each of Dr. Doppman's patients had been clearly demonstrated by localization studies, it could have been readily retrieved surgically. A properly executed exploration carries no greater risk than a laborious arteriographic study. There may be an exception in the case of an acutely ill patient when the staining therapy may serve as a stopgap measure to provide time to improve his condition before surgery. It should not, however, be used as a definitive therapy.

In conclusion, the role of the transcatheter staining therapy is limited in the management of hyperparathyroidism. While it appears sophisticated and attractive, without a pathologic diagnosis, it can be hazardous.

References

1. Wang, C.: The anatomic basis of parathyroid surgery. Ann. Surg. 183:271–275, 1976
2. Wang, C., Cope, O.: The parathyroid glands. In: Management of the Patient with Cancer, 2nd ed., edited by T.F. Nealon. Philadelphia, W.B. Saunders, 1976, pp. 256–264

Reply

John L. Doppman

It is indeed a privilege to have a surgeon of Dr. Wang's experience and stature comment on my therapeutic endeavors. Parathyroid surgery has no more qualified spokesman. And certainly whenever a radiologist ventures into the surgeon's domain, he must expect to have his techniques critically scrutinized. This is only appropriate. However, Dr. Wang has raised problems where I think none exist.

1. I agree that Gelfoam embolization is not an effective treatment for parathyroid adenomas, for precisely the reasons that Dr. Wang has enumerated. I included a summary of my embolization experience only for historical interest but thought I had clearly stated that it is an inadequate therapy.

2. It is true that hyperparathyroidism recurred in three patients early in the stain series but, in these instances, staining was accidental, very small amounts of contrast media were used, and staining persisted for less than 30 minutes. In none of the seven patients in whom staining was deliberately performed has hypercalcemia recurred, and the follow-up now extends to four years.

3. My principal issue with Dr. Wang's comments concerns the mechanism of cellular damage in staining. The results of histologic examination in animal studies have been available to me for the past year, but their publication has been delayed by a sabbatical. The findings, which were presented at the scientific session of the Society for Cardiovascular Radiology in February 1979, provide substantial histologic evidence that cellular damage from staining is severe and very likely to be permanent. Were the results of staining due solely to "ischemia resulting from arterial occlusion by the wedged catheter" as Dr. Wang suggests, hypercalcemia should have recurred within two to three months as it did in the embolization group. And to compare capillary staining with retrograde venous extravasation is to mix apples with oranges. Most attempts at adrenal ablation, to my knowledge, have been by retrograde venous perfusion. When one forcefully injects contrast media into an obstructed venous system, serial filming usually shows early rupture of a small vein and rapid deposition of a localized collection of contrast medium, displacing parenchymal elements of the target organ but not diffusely permeating them. This mechanism is different from the diffuse capillary extravasation that characterizes a wedged arterial perfusion. I would anticipate that retrograde venous extravasation would only temporarily interrupt function, as has been true of the adrenal studies to which Dr. Wang refers. This has also been our experience in a small series of patients with aldosteronomas treated by retrograde venous extravasation (Doppman, Dunnick, and Gill, unpublished observations).

4. I cannot dispute the desirability of a histologic diagnosis preceding therapy, but Dr. Wang should not minimize the morbidity of multiple operations for hyperparathyroidism, especially in hands less experienced than his. Surely the adjective "laborious" can be as aptly applied to a second or third re-exploration as to angiographic studies. The argument concerning malignancy is one to which I have called attention, but some suggestion of malignancy can usually be obtained from the arteriographic study. A small uniformly staining gland without abnormal vessels very rarely harbors malignant cells. Any gland with unusual angiographic findings is straightaway delivered to the surgeon.

New techniques invariably stimulate controversy. As the guest editor of this issue has commented elsewhere [1] radiology journals provide a service by opening their pages to such discussions. Fortunately, the ultimate role of transcatheter techniques in treating parathyroid disease will be determined by neither Dr. Wang's nor my rhetoric but by long-term follow-up of carefully controlled clinical series.

Reference

1. Athanasoulis, C.A.: Translumbar aortography revisited (letter). Am. J. Roentgenol. 133:562–563, 1979

Reply

Chiu-an Wang

I wish to extend my thanks to Dr. Doppman for his reply to my comments on his paper. I was glad to learn that all of his seven cases treated by this technique have remained cured of the disease for over four years. This record speaks well for the efficacy of the staining technique, and he and his colleagues are to be commended for these excellent results.

What remains of primary concern to me, however, is the determination of which patients with primary hyperparathyroidism should be treated by the staining technique. While I do not doubt for a moment that the staining technique has earned a place in the treatment of selected patients, in our experience, operative intervention seldom poses unsurmountable difficulties in even the most critically ill patients.

In a series of 14 patients with hyperparathyroid crisis, all but two were successfully operated upon by us, and the two patients who died were ones treated expectantly. This clearly demonstrates that surgery is to be preferred to non-operative medical treatment let alone the arduous techniques Dr. Doppman has described.

In nearly one half of our series of 20 cases of parathyroid cancer, the diagnosis was not evident at operation and was not established until the final histologic specimens were studied. Cancer of the parathyroid may resemble benign adenoma – smooth, beefy-red, firm but not stony hard – contrary to the general belief that it is always grayish-white, rock-hard, and locally invasive. While Dr. Doppman has stated that the diagnosis of parathyroid cancer can be made angiographically on the basis of a finding of abnormal blood vessels in the mass, this would seem to be more an exception than the rule.

Perhaps for patients who require a second or third operation, transcatheter staining procedure may offer an alternative therapy for hyperparathyroidism.

Reference

1. Wang, C., Guyton, S.W.: Hyperparathyroid crisis. Ann. Surg. 190:782, 1979

Final Remarks

The Treatment of Hyperparathyroidism by Transcatheter Techniques: An Endocrinologist's View

Gino V. Segre

Department of Medicine, Harvard Medical School, and Endocrine Unit, Massachusetts General Hospital, Boston, Massachusetts, USA

I read with great interest both Dr. John Doppman's report and the subsequent exchanges between Drs. Wang and Doppman. Persistent normocalcemia four years after staining in seven patients with hyperparathyroidism demonstrates that staining effectively ablates parathyroid adenomas. Potentially, this method is an important new alternative to surgery in treating this form of hyperparathyroidism. Use of this technique, however, needs to be put in clinical perspective, and the merits of the procedure must be carefully evaluated before staining can be seriously regarded as an alternative to surgery, even in treatment of parathyroid adenomas.

First, the staining technique would seem applicable only to patients in whom there is clear evidence that a single adenoma is causing the hyperparathyroidism. Dr. Doppman agrees that it is not suitable for multigland involvement, and it is inappropriate, given conventional wisdom and the absence of any pertinent evidence to the contrary, to use staining to ablate parathyroid carcinomas. Although the incidence of involvement of more than one parathyroid gland is a point of contention, it is probably fair to say that even with the benefit of localization studies, 50–60% of patients with hyperparathyroidism can be shown clearly to have a single adenoma. Thus, probably half the patients with hyperparathyroidism would be excluded from consideration for staining therapy. One must also consider that parathyroid carcinoma is frequently a pathologic diagnosis, one not apparent from either the clinical course or observations at surgery. Its occurrence, thankfully, remains quite small.

Second, after the decision is made to treat hyperparathyroidism definitively, the major surgical problem is to find the offending gland or glands. Given the benefit of a positive localization for an adenoma, competent surgeons, even those with less expert skills than Dr. Wang, should have little difficulty.

What are the relative risks and potential for cure of surgery and ablation therapy? All but one of Dr. Doppman's patients had a mediastinal tumor. In these patients, the morbidity and mortality of surgery are greatest, and the risk from ablation the smallest. However, they constitute less than 5% of patients with hyperparathyroidism. The current success rate of staining can undoubtedly be improved with greater experience, but, at present, it is probably lower than can be anticipated with surgery on an adenoma, certainly with attack on an adenoma in an identified mediastinal location.

The morbidity of neck exploration is small and the mortality approaches the risk of anesthesia in skilled hands. The potential for causing severe neurologic defects by dye injection in the thyrocervical trunk is well recognized, although the incidence of such complications is not well defined. This probably explains why only one patient with a cervical lesion appears in Dr. Doppman's initial series. Ablation of cervical lesions, even in therapeutic trials, must be undertaken cautiously even by the most skilled, like Dr. Doppman, and these trials probably should be considered by no more than a few expert radiologists in the country. In this respect, insufficient data are included to identify any role for staining therapy in cervical adenomas. Moreover, no evidence is presented to support the conclusion that the ablation technique may be particularly useful in "high-risk patients." Experience may prove that parathyroid hormone released from the glands of severely hypercalcemic patients may cause sufficient additional hypercalcemia to be contraindicated.

Address reprint requests to: G.V. Segre, M.D., Endocrine Unit, Massachusetts General Hospital, Fruit Street, Boston, MA 02114, USA

In summary, Dr. Doppman's report suggests that staining may be a particularly useful modality in the treatment of mediastinal adenomas. The limited experience with the technique, particularly with cervical lesions, does not form a study upon which changes in current therapeutic approaches can be advised. Treatment by radiologic or surgical approaches should meet the same rigorous testing that we demand from drug studies. Clearly, however, the approach shows great promise and merits further study in controlled, prospective trials with better-defined patient groups.

Splenic Embolization

Demetrios G. Spigos,[1] Walter S. Tan,[1] Martin F. Mozes,[2] Kevin Pringle,[2] and Ioulios Iossifides[3]

Departments of Radiology,[1] Surgery,[2] and Pathology,[3] University of Illinois Hospital, Chicago, Illinois, USA

Abstract. While transcatheter embolization of the spleen has shown promise in the treatment of a wide spectrum of disorders, the incidence of serious complications with this technique has limited its use as an alternative to operative splenectomy. In our institution 41 patients were treated with a modified technique involving partial splenic embolization, careful antibiotic prophylaxis, and adequate pain control. There was no mortality and only few instances of clinically significant complications: a splenic abscess in one patient, pancreatitis in one patient, severe pleural effusions in two patients, and pneumonia in five patients

Key words: Embolism, therapeutic – Catheters and catheterization – Arterial blockade – Spleen – Interventional radiology.

While transcatheter arterial embolization has gained increasing acceptance in the treatment of various conditions [1–10], the impressive successes of this new therapeutic modality have been couterbalanced by serious complications [11–15]. Splenic embolization, in particular, has been fraught with the almost-uniform development of splenic abscesses [16–23] (S. Reuter, personal communication; J. Petasnik, personal communication). In addition to abscess formation, other grave complications, such as rupture of the spleen [18], septicemia, and pneumonia [19], have hindered the use of splenic embolization as an alternative to operative splenectomy in selected cases of hypersplenism. Because of a number of modifications in the embolization technique, we have successfully performed partial splenic embolization (PSE) in 41 patients.

Materials and Methods

Patients

Since September 1976, 41 patients (25 male and 16 female, with ages ranging from nine to 75 years) have undergone PSE in our hospital. Thirty-eight of our patients underwent PSE once, while three patients were treated twice; thus, a total of 44 procedures were carried out. Embolization was performed in 17 patients because of azathioprine intolerance following renal transplantation and in seven patients on chronic hemodialysis who had evidence of hypersplenism, according to criteria described by Fisher et al. [24]. Eleven patients underwent splenic embolization as part of an ongoing prospective study designed to evaluate the role of PSE versus surgical splenectomy in renal transplantation. Five patients were treated by PSE for hypersplenism due to thalassemia major and one for bleeding esophageal varices due to splenic vein thrombosis.

Technique

Preparative measures included whole-body povidone-iodine baths the night before and as well as the morning of the embolization. Patients were begun on antibiotic prophylaxis on the morning of embolization. The first 25 patients received a combination of penicillin G and gentamicin. The last 16 patients received a one-drug prophylaxis of cefoxitin sodium (1 g intravenously every eight to 12 hours). The antibiotic prophylaxis was continued for five days.

Strict aseptic technique was observed in the angiography suite. The embolic material used in all patients was absorbable gelatin sponge cut into 2×2 mm pieces and suspended immediately before the intraarterial injection in an antibiotic solution (penicillin G 32,000 units and gentamicin 12 mg in 100 ml of normal saline). The same antibiotic solution was used instead of contrast medium for the injection of embolic particles. A femoral or axillary artery approach was used for splenic artery catheterization, and the tip of the catheter was always well advanced selectively into the splenic artery. Depending on the percentage of the spleen to be embolized 10–40 pieces of Gelfoam were injected, while the extent of infarction was monitored fluoroscopically and radiographically. No at-

---

Address reprint requests to: D.G. Spigos, M.D., Department of Radiology, University of Illinois Hospital, 840 S. Wood Street, Chicago, IL 60612, USA

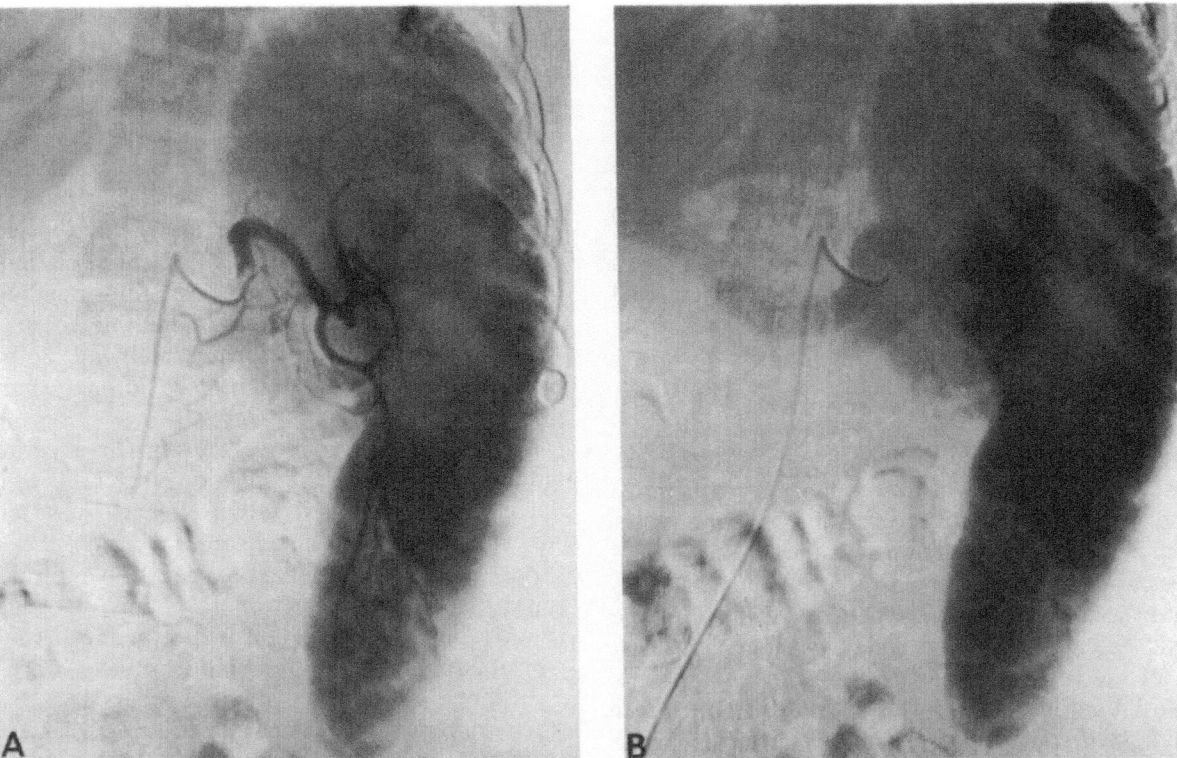

Fig. 1 A and B. Arterial phase (**A**) and venous phase (**B**) of a selective splenic arteriogram in a 21-year-old patient with thalassemia major demonstrates a grossly enlarged spleen.

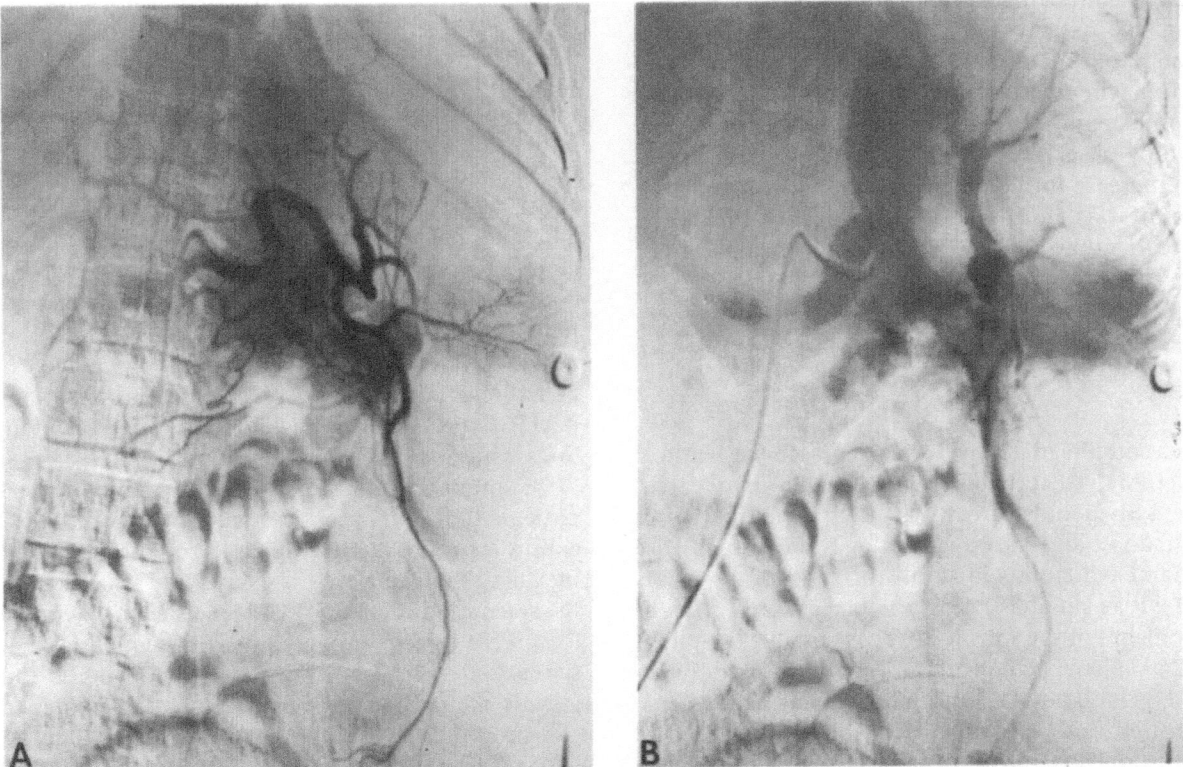

Fig. 2 A and B. Following embolization several intrasplenic branches are occluded (**A**), while in the venous phase the uninfarcted splenic parenchyma is visualized (**B**). Despite the extensive embolization (80%), the splenic vein and some of its tributaries are visualized.

tempt was made to infarct the total splenic mass; the embolization was terminated when approximately 60% of the splenic parenchyma was ablated (Figs. 1 and 2). Because the first patient experienced severe localized pain after embolization, the next five patients received 25–50 mg of meperidine hydrocholoride intravenously immediately before the embolization in addition to potent analgesics that were continued for three days. Two of these five patients also received a left intercostal block to control the early post-embolization pain. In our last 35 patients, continuous epidural anesthesia using bupicacaine hydrochloride 0.5% almost completely eliminated pain during the embolization procedure and for the following 48 hours, thus largely obviating the need for repeated doses of potent narcotics.

Results

Splenic embolization was abandoned in three patients: in one patient we were unable to catheterize the splenic artery selectively, and in two patients repeated catheterization attempts resulted in subintimal dissections. In one of our patients less than 25% infarction was obtained, in six patients 30–50% of the splenic parenchyma was ablated, in 30 patients 50–70% of the spleen was ablated, and in four patients over 70% of the spleen was infarcted. The larger the infarcted splenic mass, the more serious were the complications and adverse effects that followed this procedure. There was no mortality associated with splenic embolization in this group of 41 patients. The clinically significant complications were splenic abscess in one patient, pancreatitis in another, pleural effusion requiring thoracocentesis in two patients, and pneumonia in five patients. Adverse effects such as fever, mild paralytic ileus, and abdominal pain were commonly observed.

An increase in the platelet count and white blood cell count was noted in the first post-embolization days, with values usually returning to normal within five to 10 days.

Discussion

Various embolic materials have been used for medical splenectomy. Absorbable gelatin sponge was exclusively used in our patients as well as in the series of Owman et al. [25]. Its advantages include its ease of use and availability in sterile form. Since the pieces can be cut as small as necessary, occlusion of peripheral branches of the splenic artery is possible, resulting in partial splenic embolization. Maddison used autologous clot with good results in his patient with splenic vein thrombosis [26]. Nonabsorbable embolic agents such as polyvinyl alcohol and silastic spheres have been used successfully in the production of splenic infarctions in both humans and animals [17, 27].

Goldman et al. have advocated the use of isobutyl 2-cyanoacrylate as the occluding agent of choice since with it, occlusion of the main trunk of the splenic artery and diminution of the function of this organ can be obtained [22, 28]. When tissue adhesives, the Gianturco coil, or balloon catheters are used to occlude the main splenic artery, reconstitution of the distal branches through collaterals takes place [28, 29], and the desired effects of splenic ablation may be only temporary. Nevertheless, these methods do produce improvement in the hematologic status of patients with thrombocytopenia allowing the performance of splenectomy under more optimal conditions [18, 30].

Phillips has used direct current in experimental animals to occlude the splenic artery [31], while we have successfully used radiofrequency wave current to cause occlusion of the distal branches of the splenic artery in dogs (unpublished data).The intraarterial injection of yttrium-90 microspheres, as suggested by Ariel and Padula [32], provides yet another method for nonoperative splenic ablation.

Since no embolic material appears to satisfy all the requirements for a safe and effective splenic embolization, the choice obviously should depend on the anatomy and etiology of hypersplenism in individual patients.

Splenic embolization represents a potential alternative method to operative splenectomy when ablation of the splenic parenchyma is desired, particularly in high-risk or immunologically compromised patients in whom splenectomy carries significant morbidity and mortality [33].

Splenic embolization has been successfully used experimentally in the treatment of splenic trauma [27, 34], and has been shown to produce hematologic changes in both peripheral platelet and white cell counts [29, 35]. The changes we observed in our patients were consistent with the findings from the white cell and platelet counts documented by Owman et al. in patients who underwent splenic embolization for portal hypertension [25] and by Anderson et al. in dogs whose spleens were embolized [29].

Examination of three spleens from our series of patients (one from a patient who died from unrelated causes six months after the splenic embolization and two that were removed six days and six weeks after the splenic embolization), as well as experimental data from PSE in dogs provided us with sequential macroscopic and microscopic evidence of post-embolization splenic changes (unpublished data). Immediately after the procedure and for the following 24 hours, the entire spleen is swollen, soft, and filled with stagnating blood. The capsule is tense and considerably thinner. This appearance explains the clinical picture of severe

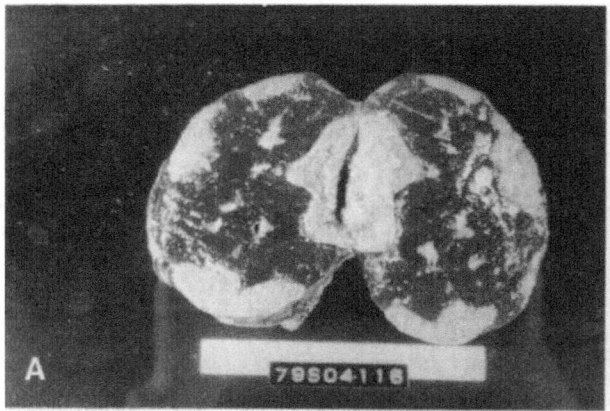
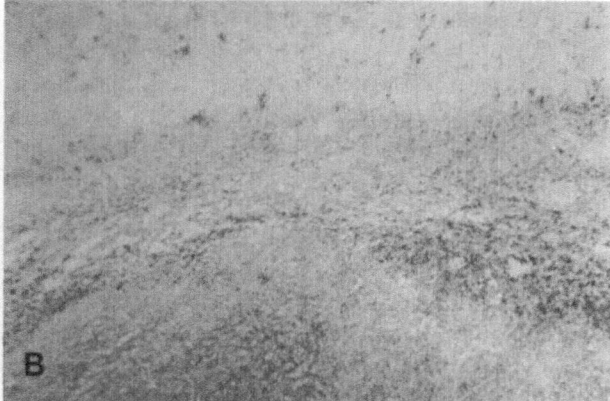

Fig. 3A and B. Macroscopic and microscopic appearance of the spleen six weeks following partial embolization. **A** Multiple subcapsular infarcts are sharply delineated, gray, soft, and irregular in shape. **B** An increasing marginal zone of granulation tissue (*center zone*) separates the infarcted area of necrosis (*upper zone*) from the normal spleen (*lower zone*).

pain and the danger of rupture during the initial post-embolization period. Microscopic evidence of organization becomes clearly manifested by the fourth post-embolization day and continues past the tenth week (unpublished data). By the sixth post-embolization week, the infarcts were well delineated from the normal parenchyma (Fig. 3), while by the sixth post-embolization month, the infarcts are sharply delineated from the noninfarcted parenchyma and were compressed and completely fibrotic. From both the human and animal experience, it appears the danger of splenic rupture is greatly minimized by the second post-embolization week.

Since 1973 when Maddison first reported a successful splenic embolization [26], a wide spectrum of splenic pathology has been treated by this technique. The use of this therapeutic modality has been advocated in the treatment of bleeding varices when other more conventional therapeutic methods have failed or manifestations of hypersplenism (e.g., thrombocytopenia or anemia) secondary to portal hypertension predominate [19–22, 25, 36, 37] as well as to control variceal bleeding in patients with splenic vein thrombosis [20, 22, 26]. The same method has also been used in patients suffering from leukemias and lymphomas [16–18, 32] (J. Petasnik, personal communication) and in patients with immune thrombocytopenic purpura [17, 18]. Berg embolized the spleen of two patients with myelofibrosis (personal communication), while Owman et al. performed embolization on a patient with polycythemia rubra vera [25]. Mozes et al. have advocated PSE in patients with azathioprine intolerance following renal transplantation [38], and Spigos et al. have used the technique in patients with hypersplenism secondary to thalassemia major (unpublished data).

In spite of consistently good short- and long-term results obtained with partial and/or sequential splenic embolizations by a number of investigators [25, 39], the overall experience with this procedure has remained negative because of complications such as splenic abscesses, septicemia, pneumonia, and splenic rupture [16–23] (S. Reuter, personal communication; J. Petasnik, personal communication). Therefore, a number of authors have suggested that this procedure be performed only as a preparative step to operative splenectomy in patients with thrombocytopenia, in order to improve their hematologic status and to facilitate operative splenectomy [18, 30].

Despite the fact that the patients in whom we performed splenic embolization represented a high-risk population who were either uremic, on continuous immunosuppression, or had markedly enlarged spleens, serious complications were rarely observed. We attribute the lack of significant complications to: (1) the differences between total and partial splenic embolizations; (2) strict aseptic technique and antibiotic prophylaxis; (3) the effective control of pain, and (4) careful pre- and post-embolization care.

Since we routinely perform only partial embolization, a portion of the splenic parenchyma with normal blood supply remains intact. While the amount of remaining splenic tissue required to provide protection from overwhelming bacterial sepsis is not known with certainty [40], it appears that 30–50% of normally vascularized splenic mass preserves the normal immune function of this organ in rats [41–43]. Pearson et al. [44] reported that some patients with splenosis showed some evidence of splenic function. Other authors have reported patients who died from overwhelming post-splenectomy sepsis in spite of significant amounts of splenic tissue demonstrated at autopsy [40, 45], thus casting doubt on the functional integrity of splenic autografts. Until some of the questions regarding the immune role of the spleen in humans have been answered with certainty, we will attempt to preserve at least 30% of normally vascularized splenic mass. Since the experimental data of Pringle et al. [32] suggest that there is some impairment of splenic function following operative partial splenectomy, it would appear advisable for patients to receive either pneumococcal vaccine prophylaxis or penicillin prophylaxis for at least 12 months.

In addition to the expected immunologic advantages, partial splenic embolization might prevent the development of splenic abscesses by preserving the normal direction of blood flow through the splenic circulation, as has been observed in our post-embolization angiograms. When the arterial flow to the spleen is completely interrupted, as occurs with total splenic embolization, there is reversal of the flow in the splenic vein [46, 47]. This reversal might cause contamination of the infarcted splenic parenchyma with bacteria carried from the gastrointestinal tract via the portal circulation.

Since the introduction of bacterially contaminated embolic particles could also result in abscess formation, antibiotic prophylaxis is also important in PSE. The bacteria most commonly isolated from splenic abscesses are Klebsiella pneumoniae, Staphylococcus epidermiditis, Clostridium perfringens, and Staphylococcus aureus [18, 19, 23]; thus, a combination of parenteral antibiotics such as penicillin-gentamycin, cephalothin sodium, or cefoxitin sodium [25, 39] should be administered. The suspension of embolic particles in antibiotic solution may also eliminate possible bacterial contamination of the embolic agents [25, 39].

Adequate pain control, which can be achieved with continuous regional (epidural) anesthesia, is important since the reduction in splinting of the abdominal, thoracic, and diaphragmatic muscles achieved allows better lung expansion and bronchial toilet [39].

References

1. Djindjian, R., Cophignon, J., Rey, A., Theron, J., Merland, J.J., Houdart, R.: Superselective arteriographic embolization by the femoral route in neuroradiology: Study of 50 cases-III, Embolization in craniocerebral pathology. Neuroradiology 6:143–153, 1973
2. Serbinenko, F.A.: Balloon catheterization and occlusion of major cerebral vessels. J. Neurosurg. 41:125–145, 1974
3. Sokoloff, J., Wickbom, I., Ingmar, X., McDonald, D., Brahme, F., Goergen, T.G., Goldberger, L.E.: Therapeutic percutaneous embolization in intractable epistaxis. Radiology 11:285–287, 1974
4. Portsmann, W., Wierny, L., Warneke, H., Gertsberger, G., Romaniuk, P.A.: Catheter closure of patent ductus arteriosus: 62 cases treated without thoracotomy. Radiol. Clin. North Am. 9:203–218, 1971
5. Rösch, J., Dotter, C.T., Brown, M.J.: Selective arterial embolization: A new method for control of acute gastrointestinal bleeding. Radiology 102:303–306, 1972
6. Reuter, S.R., Chuang, V.P., Bree, R.L.: Selective arterial embolization for control of acute gastrointestinal bleeding. Radiology 102:303–306, 1972
7. Goldman, M.L., Land, W.C., Bradley, E.L., Anderson, J.: Transcatheter therapeutic embolization in the management of massive upper gastrointestinal bleeding. Radiology 120:513–521, 1976
8. Bookstein, J.J., Naderi, M.J., Walter, J.F.: Transcatheter embolization for lower gastrointestinal bleeding. Radiology 127:345–349, 1978
9. Almgard, L.E., Fernstrom, L., Haverling, M., Ljungqvist, A.: Treatment of renal adenocarcinoma by embolic occlusion of the renal circulation. Br. J. Urol. 45:474–479, 1973
10. Miller, F.J., Mortel, R., Mann, W.J., Jahshan, A.E.: Selective arterial embolization for control of hemorrhage in pelvic malignancy: Femoral and brachial catheter approaches. Am. J. Roentgenol. 126:1028–1032, 1976
11. Woodside, J., Schwarz, H., Bergreen, P.: Peripheral embolization complicating bilateral renal infarction with Gelfoam. Am. J. Roentgenol. 126:1033–1034, 1976
12. Gang, D.L., Dole, K.B., Adelman, L.S.: Spinal cord infarction following therapeutic renal artery embolization. JAMA 237:2841–2842, 1977
13. Tegtmeyer, C.J., Smith, T.H., Shaw, A., Barwick, K.W., Kattwinkel, J.: Renal infarction: A complication of Gelfoam embolization of a hemangioendothelioma of the liver. Am. J. Roentgenol. 128:305–307, 1977
14. Bradley, E.L., Goldman, M.L.: Gastric infarction after therapeutic embolization. Surgery 79:421–424, 1976
15. Braf, Z.F., Koontz, W.W.: Gangrene of bladder: Complication of hypogastric artery embolization. Urology 9:670–671, 1977
16. Goldstein, H.M., Wallace, S., Anderson, J.H., Bree, R.L., Giantruco, C.: Transcatheter occlusion of abdominal tumors. Radiology 120:539–545, 1976
17. Castaneda-Zuniga, W.R., Hammerschmidt, D.E., Sanchez, R., Amplatz, K.: Non-surgical splenectomy. Am. J. Roentgenol. 129:805–811, 1977
18. Wholey, M.H., Chamorro, H., Rao, G., Chapman, W.: Splenic infarction and spontaneous rupture of the spleen following therapeutic embolization. Cardiovasc. Radiol. 1:249–253, 1978
19. Witte, C.L., Ovitt, T.W., Van Wyck, D.B., Witte, M.H., O'Mara, R.E., Woolfenden, J.M.: Ischemic therapy in thrombocytopenia from hypersplenism. Arch. Surg. 111:1115–1121, 1976
20. Zimmermann, H.B., Burger, K., Winter, H., Buchalik, X., Schimmelpfennig, W., Wack, R., Sielaff, F., Ihle, E.: Ausschaltung der Milzfunktion durch Milzarterien-Embolisation – Transvasale Therapie des Hypersplenismus bei Pfortaderhochdruck. Dt. Gesundh.-Wesen 34:164 166, 1979
21. Pereiras, R., Schiff, E., Barkin, J., Hutson, D.: The role of interventional radiology in diseases of the hepatobiliary system and the pancreas. Radiol. Clin. North Am. 17:555–605, 1979
22. Goldman, M.L., Philip, P.K., Sarrafizadeh, M.S., Gordon, I.J., Sarfek, J.I., Salam, A., Galambos, J.T., Powers, S.R., Smith, R.P.: Medical splenectomy by transcatheter arterial embolization with bucrylate. Presented at the 65th Annual meeting of the Radiologic Society of North America, Atlanta, Georgia, 1979
23. Trojanowski, J.Q., Harriet, T.J., Athanasoulis, C.A., Greenfield, A.J.: Hepatic and splenic infarction complications of therapeutic transcatheter embolization. Am. J. Surg. 139:272–277, 1980
24. Fisher, K.A., Mahajan, S.K., Hill, J.L., Stuart, F.P., Katz, A.I.: Prediction of azathioprine intolerance in transplant patients. Lancet 1:828–830, 1976

25. Owman, T., Lunderquist, A., Alwmark, A., Borjesson, B.: Embolization of the spleen for the treatment of splenomegaly and hypersplenism in patients with portal hypertension. Invest. Radiol. 14:457–464, 1979

26. Maddison, F.: Embolic therapy of hypersplenism. Invest. Radiol. 8:280–281, 1973

27. Guildord, W.B., Scatliff, J.H.: Transcatheter embolization of the spleen for control of splenic hemorrhage and in situ splenectomy: An experimental study using silicone spheres. Radiology 119:549–553, 1976

28. Goldman, M.L., Skorapa, V., Galambos, J.T., Oenkt, X., Jove, D.F., Silberman, M.: Intraarterial tissue adhesives for medical splenectomy in dogs. Am. J. Gastroenterol. 70:489–495, 1978

29. Anderson, J.H., Buban, A., Wallace, S., Hester, J.P., Burke, J.S.: Transcatheter splenic arterial occlusion: An experimental study in dogs. Radiology 125:95–102, 1977

30. Levy, J.M., Wasserman, P., Pitha, N.: Presplenectomy transcatheter occlusion of the splenic artery. Arch. Surg. 114:198–199, 1979

31. Philipps, J.F.: Transcatheter electrocoagulation of blood vessels. Invest. Radiol. 8:295–304, 1973

32. Ariel, I.M., Padula, G.: Irradiation of the spleen by the intraarterial administration of yttrium-90 microspheres in patients with malignant lymphoma. Cancer 31:90–96, 1973

33. Bergin, J.J., Zuck, T.F., Millder, R.E.: Compelling splenectomy in medically compromised patients. Ann. Surg. 178:761–768, 1973

34. Chuang, V.P., Reuter, S.R.: Selective arterial embolization for the control of traumatic splenic bleeding. Invest. Radiol. 10:18–24, 1975

35. Chuang, V.P., Reuter, S.R.: Experimental diminution of splenic function by selective embolization of the splenic artery. Surg. Gynecol. Obstet. 140:715–720, 1975

36. Bucheler, E., Thalen, M., Schirmer, G., Schulz, D., Frommhold, H., Siedeck, M., Kaufer, C.: Katheterembolisation der Milzarterien zum Stopp der akuten Varizenblutung. Fortschr. Röntgenstr. 1220:224–229, 1975

37. Papadimitriou, J., Tritakis, C., Karatzas, G., Papaioannou, A.: Treatment of hypersplenism by embolus placement in the splenic artery. Lancet 2:1268–1269, 1976

38. Mozes, M., Spigos, D., Jonasson, O., Thomas, P.: Transcatheter partial splenic embolization for azathioprine intolerance in renal transplant recipients. Transplant. Proceed. 11:45–48, 1979

39. Spigos, D.G., Jonasson, O., Mozes, M., Capek, V.: Partial splenic embolization in the treatment of hyperplenism. Am. J. Roentgenol. 132:777–782, 1979

40. Rice, H.M., James, P.D.: Ectopic splenic tissue: Failed to prevent fatal pneumococcal septicaemia after splenectomy for trauma. Lancet 1:565–566, 1980

41. Van Wyck, D.B., Witte, M.H., Witte, C.L., Thies, A.C.: Critical splenic mass for survival from experimental pneumococcemia. J. Surg. Res. 28:14–17, 1980

42. Coil, J.A., Dickerman, J.P., Horner, S.R., Chalmer, B.J.: Pulmonary infection in splenectomized mice: Protection by splenic remnant. J. Surg. Res. 28:18–22, 1980

43. Pringle, K.C., Rowley, D.M., Burrington, J.D.: Immunological response in splenectomized and partially splenectomized rats. J. Pcd. Surg. (in press)

44. Pearson, H.A., Johnston, D., Smith, K.A., Touloukian, R.J.: The born-again spleen: Return of splenic function after splenectomy for trauma. N. Engl. J. Med. 298:1389–1392, 1978

45. Gopal, V., Bisno, A.L.: Fulminant pneumococcal infection in "normal asplenic hosts." Arch. Intern. Med. 137:1526–1530,

46. Witte, C.L., Witte, M.H., Renert, W., O'Mara, R.E., Lilien, D.L.: Splenic artery ligation in selected patients with hepatic cirrhosis and in sprague Dawley rats. Surg. Gynecol. Obstet. 142:1–12, 1976

47. Tsapogas, J.J., Peabody, R.A., Karmody, A.M., Chuntrasakul, C., Goussous, H., Eckert, C.: Patho-physiological changes following ischemia of the spleen. Ann. Surg. 178:179–185, 1973

Comment

Splenic Embolization: A Surgeon's View

A. Benedict Cosimi

Department of Surgery, Harvard Medical School and Massachusetts General Hospital, Boston, Massachusetts, USA

Transcatheter arterial embolization to decrease or ablate splenic function is an attractive approach to hypersplenism, particularly in the immunocompromised host. Not only may the morbidity and mortality associated with surgical splenectomy be avoided, but the non-infarcted spleen may continue to provide those immunologic functions essential for the prevention

Address reprint requests to: A.B. Cosimi, M.D., Department of Surgery, Massachusetts General Hospital, Fruit Street, Boston, MA 02114, USA

of overwhelming bacterial sepsis, which has been observed in 2–3% of splenectomized children and occasionally in adults as well. Previous experimental and clinical reports, however, have emphasized the frequent occurrence of splenic abscesses or rupture as serious potential consequences of the embolization procedure and, thus, have advised limiting this approach only to patients in whom the risk of an operative procedure is felt to be unacceptable.

Spigos and his colleagues have continued a carefully designed evaluation of the transcatheter approach and now report its successful performance in 41 of 44 patients in whom it was attempted. By adhering to a strict protocol including use of local and systemic antibiotics, careful aseptic techniques, and effective post-embolization nursing care and pain control to avoid muscle splinting and pulmonary morbidity, they have reported no fatal complications in this series. While significant morbidity was noted in nine patients, there was, however, only one abscess. Milder side effects, including fever, ileus, and abdominal pain, apparently occurred quite frequently. Using this protocol, therefore, these investigators have reduced the mortality and morbidity rates to a level at least comparable with what has been reported following surgical splenectomy.

The most important key to this group's success, however, would appear to be the emphasis on partial rather than total splenic arterial embolization. The authors point out that the precisely desired amount of splenic parenchyma may not be infarcted during the initial attempt with the selective embolization procedure but that the technique can be performed safely and effectively in the same patient on repeated occasions. Although the exact percentage is yet to be determined, apparently if 70% or less of the splenic mass is infarcted the risk of subsequent splenic abscess or rupture is markedly reduced while hematologic improvement usually occurs. The suggestion that, following more extensive infarction, reversal of splenic vein blood flow contributes to the risk of infection

by transport of gastrointestinal tract flora to the spleen is a logical assumption that awaits confirmation from further investigations.

A perhaps even more important benefit of partial embolization is that by this means the true goal of treatment for hypersplenism, which should be to reduce but not totally eliminate splenic function, can be achieved. Whether, indeed, preservation of splenic parenchyma by this technique will provide the immunologic function necessary to prevent serious postsplenectomy infectious complications remains to be determined in randomized, prospective trials such as these investigators have already begun. It will be of interest, as well, to define in these studies in transplant patients whether preservation of a portion of the spleen negates the beneficial effect on allograft survival which has been observed by some groups following surgical splenectomy.

Despite these limitations in our understanding of the long-term immunologic consequences, it is clear from the experience already gained by this group that partial splenic embolization using the carefully defined techniques they have reported is a procedure that can be safely and successfully extended to increasing numbers of patients with hypersplenism. As more data become available, it may become evident that the immunologic benefits of partial infarction as opposed to surgical splenectomy may be the most significant difference between the procedures.

Transcatheter Embolization versus Vasopressin Infusion for the Control of Arteriocapillary Gastrointestinal Bleeding

Arthur C. Waltman

Department of Radiology, Harvard Medical School and Massachusetts General Hospital, Boston, Massachusetts, USA

Abstract. The transcatheter method appropriate for use in the control of arteriocapillary gastrointestinal bleeding is a point of controversy. Intraarterial vasopressin infusion, which has been performed in more than 500 patients at the Massachusetts General Hospital, has achieved control in 90% of patients actively bleeding from the stomach and colon. In view of the severity of hemorrhage and associated illnesses in these patients, the complication rate associated with this method was low. Intraarterial vasopressin infusions were ineffective in pyloroduodenal and postoperative bleeding sites and hemorrhage from abscesses. While embolization can control bleeding in these areas, complications have been shown despite precise selective catheter placement. Because of catheterization difficulties and the permanency of the vascular occlusion, embolization is reserved for patients in whom surgical intervention would be associated with extreme risks.

Key words: Gelfoam – Embolism, therapeutic – Arteries, therapeutic blockade – Catheters and catheterization – Vasopressin – Gastrointestinal tract, hemorrhage – Interventional radiology.

Following the successful application of angiography in the localization of gastrointestinal bleeding sites, investigators attempted to control hemorrhage using therapeutic angiographic techniques. Two methods have been used: (1) the intraarterial infusion of vasopressin [1] (and, more recently, its low-dose-rate sas thera infusion [2]) and (2) transcatheter embolization [3, 4]. The method of choice remains in dispute. In this paper an attempt is made to present a rational approach to the selection of the most appropriate angiographic method in various sites.

Stomach

Localization of bleeding originating from the stomach and distal esophagus is usually established by endoscopy with confirmation of continued bleeding achieved by nasogastric aspiration. Bleeding sites in the stomach and distal esophagus are supplied by the branches of the left gastric artery. Selective arteriography shows focal points of extravasation in 60% of cases. Left gastric arterial infusion of vasopressin at 0.2 unit per minute controls bleeding in 82% of cases (Fig. 1) [5]. If bleeding is not controlled, the infusion dose rate may be increased to 0.3 or 0.4 unit per minute and the effect confirmed with repeat arteriography. The rate of recurrent bleeding following control with vasopressin is 16% [6, 7].

In approximately 40% of patients bleeding from erosive or alcoholic gastritis, the arteriogram shows nonspecific hyperemia of the gastric wall without contrast extravasation. In these cases, the decision to infuse vasopressin into the left gastric artery is based on endoscopic findings and the failure to show other bleeding sites on splenic and hepatic arterial injections. At times bleeding sites in the stomach and distal esophagus may be supplied by a dominant right gastric, short gastric, or gastric arteries having a common origin with the inferior phrenic arteries. The use of the loop technique allows selective catheterization of the left gastric artery in 95% of cases, although anatomic variations, such as those mentioned above, may make this task more difficult [8, 9]. When the catheter tip cannot be placed in the left gastric artery, vasopressin may be infused in the celiac axis with an expected bleeding control rate of 65% [5].

Address reprint requests to: A.C. Waltman, M.D., Department of Radiology, Massachusetts General Hospital, Fruit Street, Boston, MA 02114, USA

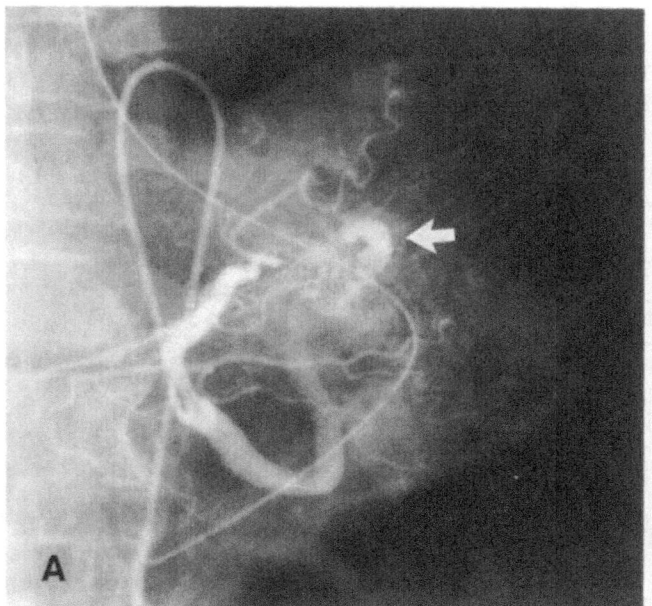
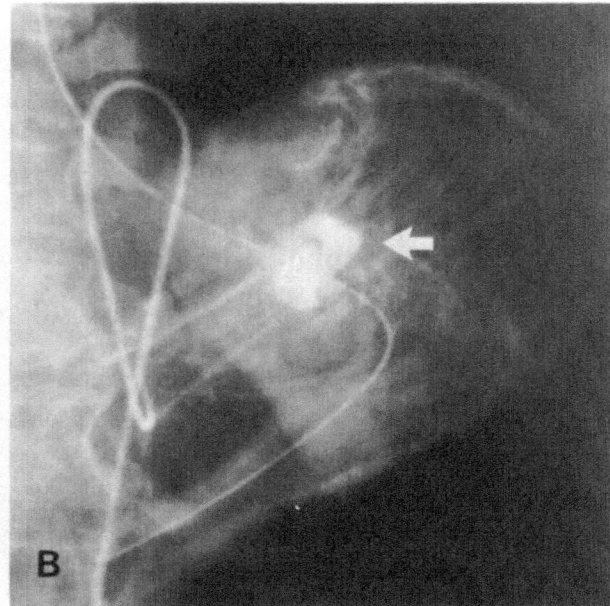
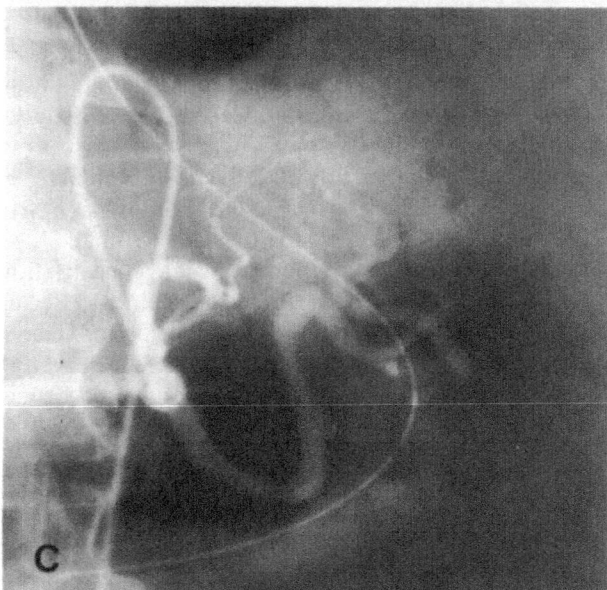

Fig. 1 A–C. Massive bleeding from gastritis controlled with vasopressin in an elderly man who had recent abdominal surgery.
A Arterial phase of left gastric artery injection showing extravasation in the proximal stomach (*arrow*).
B Venous phase of left gastric arteriogram showing accumulation of contrast material (*arrow*) in the proximal stomach.
C Control arteriogram following twenty minutes of vasopressin infusion in the left gastric artery at a rate of 0.2 unit per minute shows no extravasation. The bleeding was also clinically controlled.

Fig. 2 A–D. Massive bleeding from gastritis controlled with embolization in a middle-aged woman who had recent major abdominal surgery.
A Selective left gastric arteriogram. Early arterial phase shows accumulation of contrast in the mid portion of the lesser curvature of the stomach (*arrow*).
B Later arterial phase from the left gastric arteriogram demonstrates massive contrast extravasation in the stomach (*arrows*).
C Selective control left gastric arteriogram showing reduction in the amount of contrast extravasation from the bleeding point in the stomach following infusion of vasopressin at 0.4 unit per minute. Although the bleeding is reduced arteriographically, it would, however, be unusual for clinical control to be established under these circumstances.
D Left gastric arteriogram following embolization of the left gastric artery with small strips of Gelfoam demonstrates control of the bleeding. The bleeding was also clinically controlled.

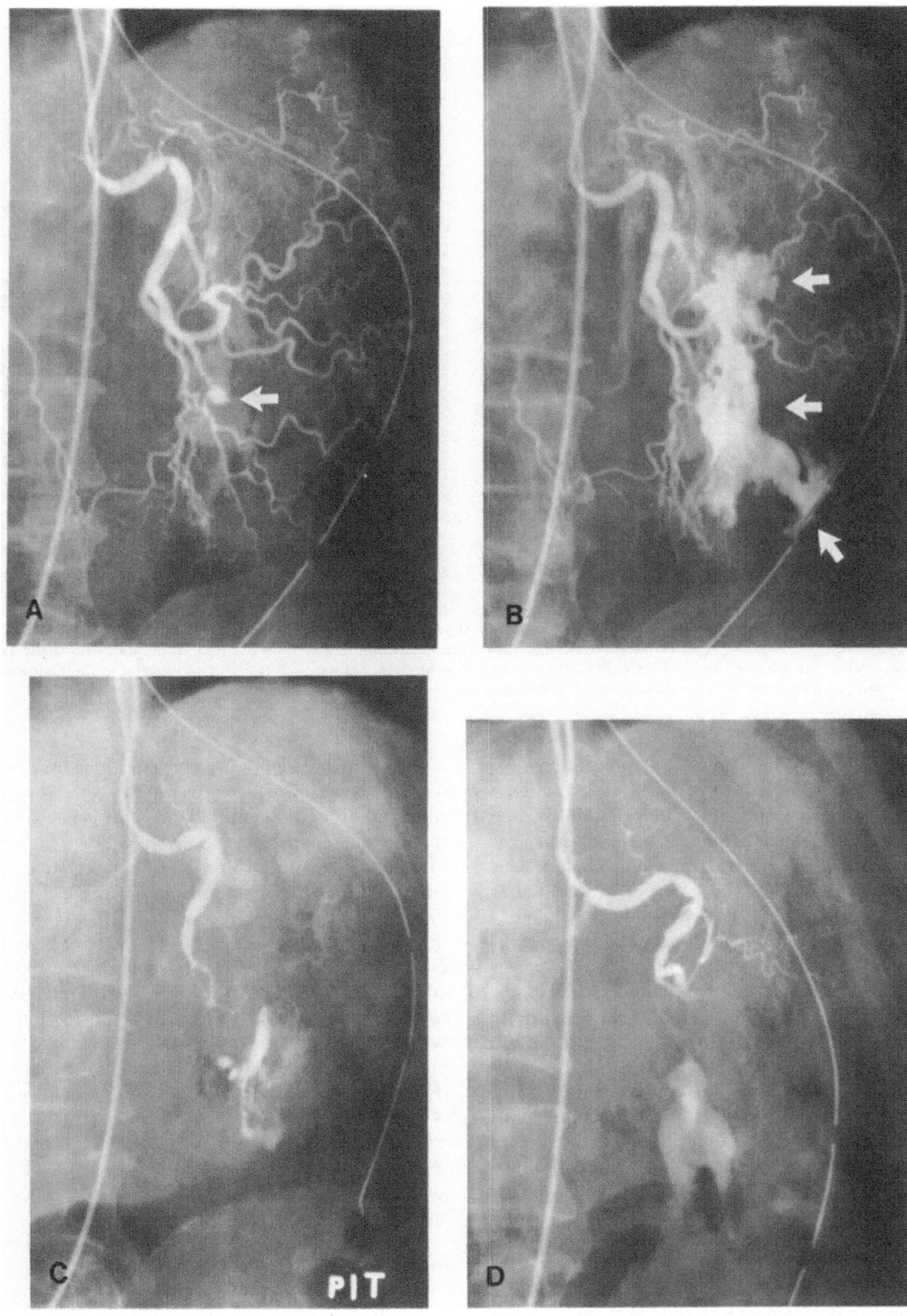

Fig. 2 A–D

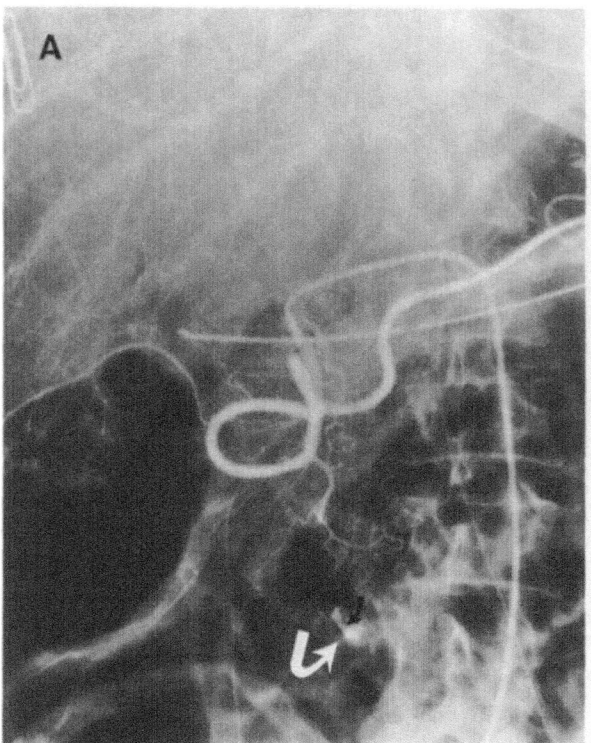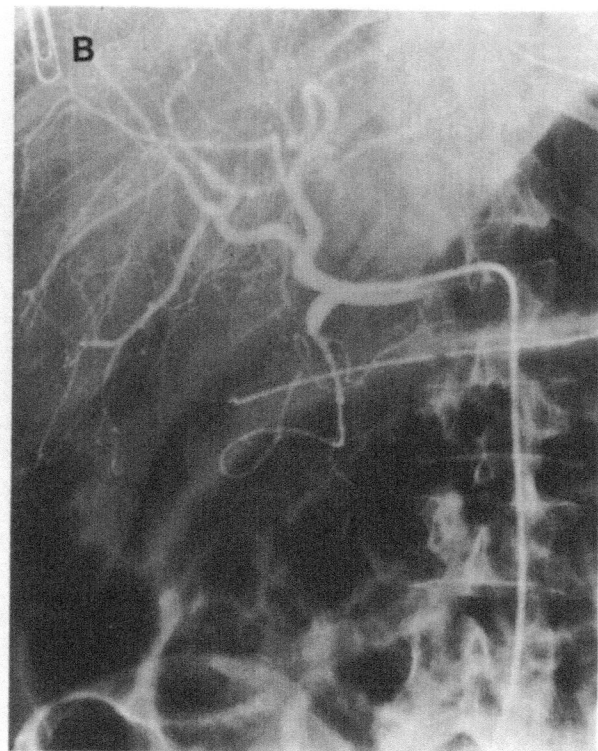

Fig. 3A and B. Bleeding from a duodenal ulcer controlled with vasopressin in a young man who had experienced the sudden onset of upper gastrointestinal bleeding. **A** Selective gastroduodenal arteriogram demonstrates extravasation from branches of the superior pancreaticoduodenal artery (*curved arrows*). **B** Control arteriogram following twenty minutes of vasopressin infusion in the gastroduodenal artery at 0.3 unit per minute shows no extravasation. The bleeding was also clinically controlled.

Vasopressin infusion is favored over embolization because of the diffuse nature of bleeding in patients with gastric stress bleeding and erosive and alcoholic gastritis. Transcatheter embolization with surgical gelatin is reserved for patients in whom vasopressin fails to control bleeding (Fig. 2). For transcatheter embolization, selective catheter positioning is mandatory. Reflux of embolic material is a potential complication that may result in ischemic injury to the spleen, pancreas, or liver. In addition, if embolization is not peripheral but results in proximal occlusion of the left gastric artery, collateral flow will reconstitute the distal non-obstructed bleeding branch, and hemorrhage will continue. Also, previous extensive gastric surgery increases the risk of gastric infarction. With these limitations, embolization in selected patients may be undertaken by experienced vascular radiologists.

Duodenum

Vasopressin is less effective in pyloroduodenal bleeding than in gastric mucosal hemorrhage. The reported control rate in pyloroduodenal bleeding is 31%, with recurrent bleeding in 33% (Fig. 3) [10].

There are three possible explanations for this poor response to vasopressin infusion. First, the dual blood supply to the duodenum from the celiac axis and superior mesenteric arteries, which allows the reversal of blood flow within this loop of the pancreaticoduodenal arcades, may make therapy based on occluding flow from one side of the loop ineffective [11]. Second, the inflammatory reaction associated with penetrating ulcers may play a part in decreasing vasopressin's effectiveness. Vasopressin causes not only vascular constriction but also bowel wall contraction; both actions are responsible for the reduction of arterial blood flow to the bowel wall and the bleeding site [12]. When, because of associated inflammation, there is impairment of bowel and vessel contraction, vasopressin is less effective. Third, pyloroduodenal bleeding frequently arises from large vessels, such as the gastroduodenal artery, which do not constrict in response to vasopressin.

Patients with endoscopically demonstrated pyloroduodenal bleeding who are reasonably good surgical candidates do not need control with angiographic methods. Surgical treatment offers a more satisfactory approach because it not only controls bleeding but also manages the physiologic basis of the ulcer dis-

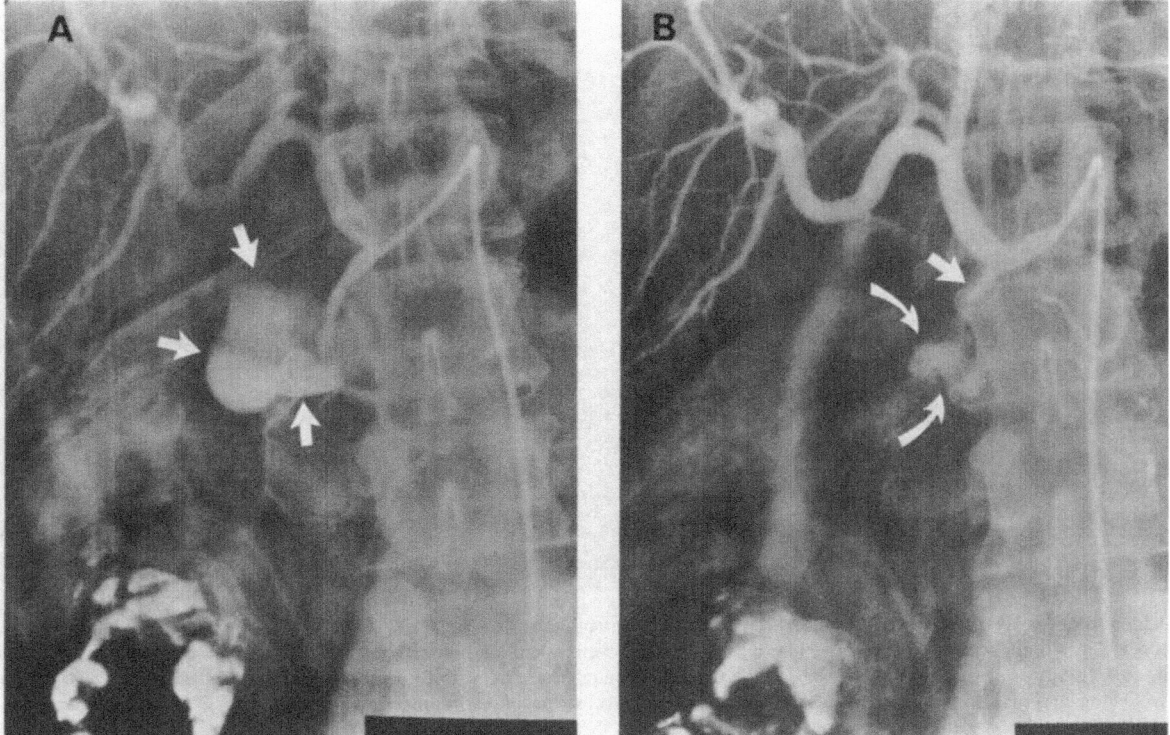

Fig. 4A and B. Massive bleeding from a duodenal ulcer controlled with embolization in a young man who had multiple abdominal surgical procedures for regional enteritis. **A** Selective gastroduodenal arteriogram demonstrating massive extravasation from the gastroduodenal artery (*arrows*). **B** Control arteriogram following infusion of a 50% isobutyl 2-cyanoacrylate and ethiodol mixture showing occlusion of the gastroduodenal artery (*arrow*) as well as opacified embolic material within the ulcer crater and the gastroduodenal artery and its branches (*curved arrows*). The bleeding was clinically controlled.

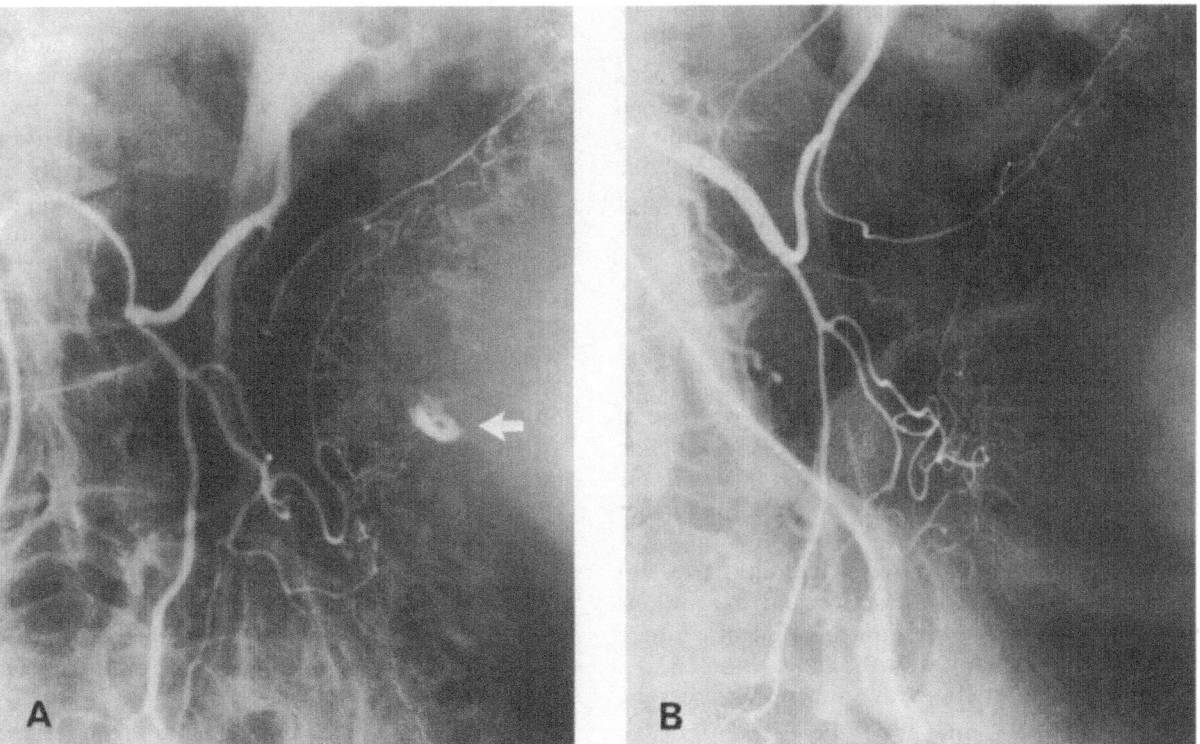

Fig. 5A and B. Massive, painless rectal hemorrhage of recent onset controlled with vasopressin in an elderly man. **A** Selective inferior mesenteric arteriogram shows extravasation from branches in the area of the descending colon (*arrow*). **B** Control arteriogram following twenty minutes of intraarterial vasopressin infusion in the inferior mesenteric artery at 0.2 unit per minute shows no extravasation. The bleeding was clinically controlled.

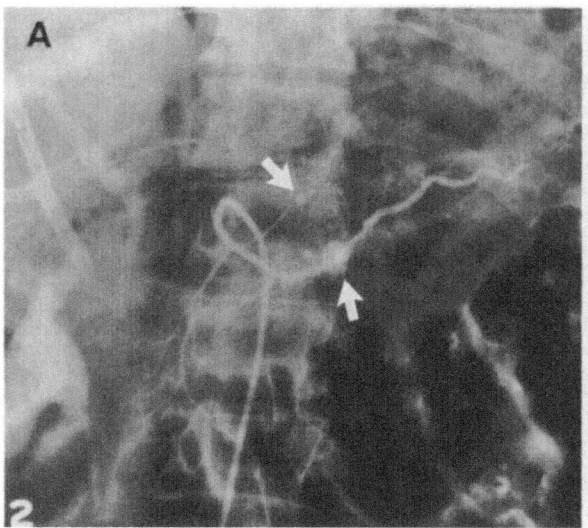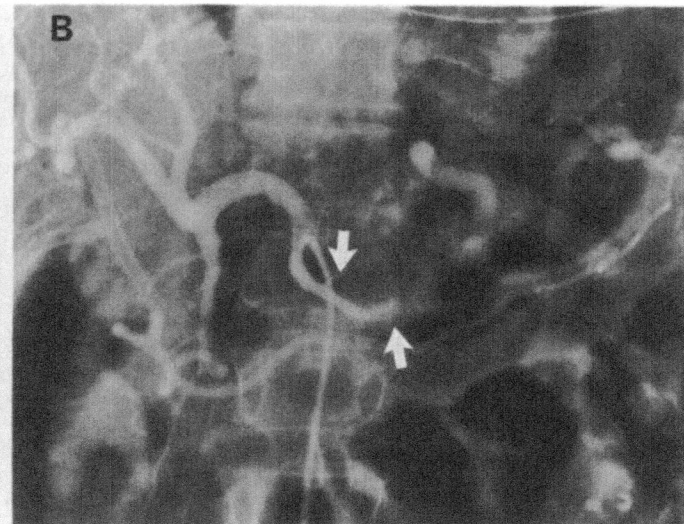

Fig. 6A and B. Massive upper gastrointestinal hemorrhage controlled by the selective embolization of the dorsal pancreatic artery in an elderly man with recent biliary surgery and subsequent development of hemorrhagic pancreatitis. **A** Selective dorsal pancreatic arteriogram demonstrating multiple aneurysms of the transverse pancreatic artery and intrapancreatic arteries (*arrows*). **B** Control arteriogram following embolization of the dorsal pancreatic artery with strips of Gelfoam showing occlusion of the artery and its major branches (*arrows*). The bleeding was controlled clinically.

ease. For patients who are poor surgical risks or in whom, because of associated illness, surgery is not desirable, vasopressin infusion may be attempted and if ineffective, transcatheter embolization can then be carried out (Fig. 4). The difficulties with embolization include the selective catheter placement and the need to achieve occlusion of large vessels both proximal and distal to the bleeding site. Techniques utilizing balloon catheters for precise introduction of embolic materials and prevention of reflux of emboli are useful [3], as are mechanical devices, such as detachable balloons, steel coils, and the tissue adhesives [13].

Small Bowel and Colon

Localization of bleeding sites in patients with rectal bleeding is difficult with endoscopy. Radionuclide blood-pool labels have recently shown promise for the selection of actively bleeding patients for further angiographic studies [14].

In patients with massive rectal bleeding, arteriography remains the most attractive and expeditious means of localizing the bleeding site and also offers the potential for therapy with the same catheter.

Vasopressin infusion in the superior mesenteric artery controls bleeding in 90% of patients with bleeding colonic diverticula (Fig. 5) [15]. In addition to vasoconstriction, vasopressin results in bowel contraction, which cleans the bowel of retained blood products. During the vasopressin infusion, bowel

preparation is begun so that if surgery proves necessary, it can be performed in a prepared patient on a semi-elective basis rather than as an urgent procedure.

Embolization of bleeding sites in the mesenteric vascular bed has not been proved safe since bowel infarction and/or bowel wall stricture have been reported as sequellae of embolization of mesenteric arterial branches [16]. We have superselectively embolized a small branch of a jejunal artery in two patients with bleeding from anastomotic ulcers following gastrojejunostomy, achieving control of the bleeding in both cases. We have also performed Gelfoam embolization of the superior hemorrhoidal artery for rectal bleeding. However, embolization of the remaining mesenteric arterial branches cannot be considered safe on the basis of currently available data.

In other causes of gastrointestinal hemorrhage, including hematobilia and pancreatitis with hemorrhage from the pancreatic duct and erosion of large vascular structures such as the gastroduodenal, hepatic, or splenic arteries (Fig. 6), vasopressin infusion is ineffective, and permanent occlusion of the bleeding vessel is necessary. The choice of materials in such cases is discussed elsewhere in this issue.

Complications

Complications of vasopressin infusion performed for control of gastrointestinal bleeding in 550 patients have been reviewed by Greenfield et al. [17]. These include electrolyte abnormalities, excessive peripheral vasoconstriction, and cardiac arrthythmias. There was no difference in the complication rate between systemic and intraarterial infusions. In light of the severity of the disease in these patients and their hemodynamic instability, this complication rate was remarkably low.

Experience with transcatheter embolization in the gastrointestinal arteries is limited, and the complications may prove unacceptably high. Improvements in technique and asepsis may reduce these complications. However, on the basis of data currently available it may be concluded that the liberal use of embolization will result in a higher complication rate without achieving better control than can be obtained with intraarterial vasopressin infusions. Embolization should be reserved for patients at high risk for surgery and should be carried out only after the potential complications are balanced against the risk of an operative intervention.

In summary, we first approach the treatment of arteriocapillary gastrointestinal bleeding by the intraarterial infusion of vasopressin. If this fails to control bleeding, we consider superselective embolization of the left gastric and gastroduodenal arterial branches. We avoid embolization of mesenterial arterial branches since the safety of this approach has not been demonstrated.

References

1. Alfidi, R.J., Caldwell, D.E., Tarar, R., Klein, H.J., Hermann, R.E., Weakley, F.L., Turnbull, R.B., Jr.: Recognition of angiosurgical detection of arteriovenous malformations of the bowel. Ann. Surg. 174:573–582, 1971
2. Widrich, W.C., Johnson, W.C., Robbins, A.H., Nabseth, D.C.: Esophagogastric variceal hemorrhage. Arch. Surg. 113:1331–1338, 1978
3. Eisenberg, H., Steer, M.L.: The nonoperative treatment of massive pyloroduodenal hemorrhage by retracted autologous clot embolization. Surgery 79:414–420, 1976
4. Bookstein, J.J., Naderi, M.J., Walter, J.F.: Transcatheter embolization for lower gastrointestinal bleeding. Radiology 127:345–349, 1978
5. Athanasoulis, C.A., Baum, S., Waltman, A.C., Ring, E.J., Imbembo, A., Vander Salm, T.J.: Control of acute gastric mucosal hemorrhage: Intra-arterial infusion of posterior pituitary extract. N. Engl. J. Med. 290:597–603, 1974
6. Athanasoulis, C.A., Waltman, A.C., Novelline, R.A., Krudy, A.G., Sniderman, K.W.: Angiography: Its contribution to the emergency management of gastrointestinal hemorrhage. Rad. Clin. North Am. 14:265–280, 1976
7. Conn, H.O., Ramsby, G.R., Storer, E.H., Mutchnik, M.G., Joshi, P.H., Phillips, M.M., Cohen, C.A., Field, G.N., Petroski, D.: Intraarterial vasopressin in the treatment of upper gastrointestinal hemorrhage: A prospective, controlled clinical trial. Gastroenterology 68:211–221, 1975
8. Waltman, A.C., Courey, W.R., Athanasoulis, C.A., Baum, S.: Technique for left gastric artery catheterization. Radiology 109:732–734, 1973
9. Athanasoulis, C.A., Baum, S., Waltman, A.C., Smith, J.C., Widrich, W.C.: Blood supply of the stomach and angiographic management of gastric bleeding: Practical considerations. Presented at the 60th Scientific Assembly and Annual Meeting of the Radiological Society of North America, Chicago, December 1–6, 1974, p. 142
10. Waltman, A.C., Greenfield, A.J., Novelline, R.A., Athanasoulis, C.A.: Pyloroduodenal bleeding and intraarterial vasopressin: Clinical results. Am. J. Roentgenol. 133:643–646, 1979
11. Ring, E.J., Oleaga, J.A., Freiman, D., Husted, J.W., Waltman, A.C., Jr., Baum, S.: Pitfalls in angiographic management of hemorrhage: Hemodynamic considerations. Am. J. Roentgenol. 129:1007–1013, 1977
12. Athanasoulis, C.A., Waltman, A.C., Novelline, R.A., Krudy, A.G., Sniderman, K.W.: Angiography: Its contribution to emergency management of GI bleeding. Rad. Clin. North Am. 14:265–280, 1976
13. Reuter, S.R.: Embolization of gastrointestinal hemorrhage (Editorial). Am. J. Roentgenol. 133:557–558, 1979
14. Winzelberg, G.G., McKusick, K.A., Strauss, H.W., Waltman, A.C., Greenfield, A.J.: Evaluation of gastrointestinal bleeding by red blood cells labeled in vivo with technetium-99m. J. Nucl. Med. 20:1080–1086, 1979
15. Athanasoulis, C.A., Baum, S., Rösch, J., Waltman, A.C., Ring, E.J., Smith, J.C., Jr., Sugarbaker, E., Wood, W.: Mesenteric arterial infusions of vasopressin for hemorrhage from colonic diverticulosis. Am. J. Surg. 129:212–216, 1975
16. Mitty, H.A., Efremidis, S., Keller, J.R.: Colonic stricture after transcatheter embolization for diverticular bleeding. Am. J. Roentgenol. 133:519–521, 1979
17. Greenfield, A.J., Waltman, A.C., Athanasoulis, C.A., Novelline, R.A., Dedrick, C.G.: Vasopressin in control of gastrointestinal hemorrhage: Complications of selective intra-arterial vs. systemic infusions (abstract). Gastroenterology 76, Part 2:1144, 1979

Comment

Embolization versus Vasopressin Infusion in Gastrointestinal Bleeding

Joseph J. Bookstein

Department of Radiology, University Hospital, San Diego, California, USA

Dr. Waltman is to be commended for his attempt to define the roles of transcatheter embolization or infusion and to rationalize the use of transcatheter techniques.

In our group, the use of transcatheter methods relative to each other and operative therapy is based on the following principles:

1. Emergency operation for gastrointestinal hemorrhage is associated with greater mortality and morbidity than elective operation or successful transcatheter hemostasis [1–3]. The differences increase in older patients and in lower gastrointestinal bleeding. For example, the mortality following emergency operation for upper gastrointestinal hemorrhage in patients under age 60 was 8%, versus 2% for early elective operation. In the age group over 60, there was a 25% mortality rate for emergency operation and a 14% mortality rate for early elective operation [1]. Thus, in elderly patients or other high-risk groups, strenous efforts at transcatheter therapy are warranted in an effort to delay or completely obviate operation.

2. Even elective operation is associated with considerable morbidity, particularly if gastrectomy or subtotal colectomy is required. Therefore, when gastrectomy or colectomy is the alternative to transcatheter hemostasis, transcatheter hemostatic methods that provide the best chance of permanent control are used.

3. Transcatheter hemostatic methods are most effective when the underlying tissues are relatively healthy and the inciting hemorrhagic factor is discontinuous. Examples of such conditions are a Mallory-Weiss tear or colonic diverticulosis, while examples of the contrary include duodenal or gastric ulcer.

Hemorrhage due to these latter conditions is ordinarily treated operatively.

4. In the treatment of arteriocapillary bleeding, the intraarterial administration of vasopressin is more effective than is intravenous administration. The intravenous and intraarterial routes are about equally effective in the treatment of variceal bleeding.

5. Vasopressin infusion is associated with frequent problems and complications. There is a significant incidence of severe peripheral vasoconstriction or cardiac ischemia, and vasopressin is relatively contraindicated in patients with coronary artery insufficiency. The prolonged intraarterial catheter position imposes significant nursing problems in postangiographic management: an infusion must be continued at all times to maintain catheter patency, the patient must be relatively immobile to prevent catheter dislocation, portable films are often required to assure proper catheter position, and the puncture site must be attended to prevent infection or bleeding.

6. On the other hand, embolization enables prompt withdrawal of the catheter. The patient then requires observation primarily for signs of ischemic injury to the bowel or recurrent hemorrhage. Embolization, however, requires at least subselective catheter placement, which cannot always be achieved, and there is significant risk of ischemic sequelae. The incidence of ischemic injury may be minimized by injecting the least number of emboli required to gain hemostasis; the degree of hemostasis achieved is usually determined fluoroscopically via small injections of contrast medium after each embolus.

7. A variety of embolic agents are available, enabling custom tailoring for specific clinical situations. If only transient occlusion of small vessels is required, as in a Mallory-Weiss tear, autologous clot is suitable. If more permanent obstruction of medium-sized arteries is desired, as in diverticular hemorrhage, Gelfoam, Ivalon, or coils may be used.

Address reprint requests to: J.J. Bookstein, M.D., Department of Radiology, University Hospital, 225 W. Dickinson St., San Diego, CA 92103, USA

8. Abundant collateral pathways exist in the stomach and moderate collateral potential exists in the small and large bowel, making embolization generally tolerable when used with moderation. Embolization probably promotes hemostasis by decreasing mean and pulsatile perfusion pressures rather than by completely blocking the hemorrhaging vascular bed.

With these principles in mind, we use intraarterial vasopressin infusion initially in the management of hemorrhage from a Mallory-Weiss tear or gastritis, and in gastric or duodenal ulcer if subselective catheterization appears to be difficult. The dose is ordinarily 0.2 units per minute. The infusion is continued at least 24 hours in gastritis because this condition is often slow to respond. In other conditions, infusion is abandoned if hemostasis is not achieved after 20 minutes, and subselective catheterization is attempted in preparation for embolization. If subselective catheterization is difficult or impossible, vasopressin is tried again at 0.3–0.4 units per minute. We avoid the use of vasopressin in patients with coronary artery disease.

In diverticular hemorrhage, the rate of failure or recurrent hemorrhage after intraarterial vasopressin has been about 50% in my experience. For this reason, I often prefer embolization as the primary mode of therapy. Our group has achieved permanent control in each of seven embolized cases of diverticular hemorrhage. One of these patients developed postembolic transmural sigmoid infarction and required a partial colectomy on a semi-emergency basis.

If subselective catheterization is impossible, diverticular hemorrhage is treated with intraarterial vasopressin infusion. Indeed, some members of our group still consider vasopressin the treatment of choice. If hemorrhage is controlled, colectomy is not advised unless hemorrhage recurs.

Embolization has been applied in three patients with recurrent gastrointestinal hemorrhage from angiodysplasias; two of the lesions were in the ascending colon, and one was in the stomach. In a fourth case with Osler-Weber syndrome, a large jejunal arteriovenous malformation was embolized. Each case benefitted, although recurrent bleeding occurred after weeks or months.

In summary, the major aim of transcatheter therapy is to avoid emergency operation, and often to obviate operation altogether. Various principles will influence the choice between vasopressin infusion or embolization. From a practical standpoint, however, the choice is frequently dictated by failure of one technique or the other, contraindications to vasopressin, or inability to catheterize a bleeding vessel subselectively. The angiographer, therefore, cannot afford to depend on one method only. In the appropriate circumstances, he must be prepared to apply either or both methods.

References

1. Schiller, K.F.R., Truelove, S.C., Williams, D.G.: Haematemesis and melaena, with special reference to factors influencing the outcome. Br. Med. J. 2:7–14, 1970
2. McGinn, F.P.: Effects of haemorrhage upon surgical operations. Br. J. Surg. 63:742–746, 1976
3. Localio, S.A., Stahl, W.M.: Diverticular disease of the alimentary tract. Curr. Probl. Surg. December, 1967
4. Bookstein, J.J., Naderi, M.J., Walter, J.F.: Transcatheter embolization for lower gastrointestinal bleeding. Radiology 127:345–349, 1978

Transhepatic Embolization of Varices

Warren C. Widrich,[1] Alan H. Robbins,[1] and Donald C. Nabseth[2]

Departments of Radiology,[1] and Surgery,[2] Boston Veterans Administration Medical Center and Tufts University School of Medicine, Boston, Massachusetts, USA

Abstract. Percutaneous transhepatic embolization of varices (PTEV) has proved to be effective in the control variceal bleeding, particularly in Child's Class C Category patients whose bleeding was not adequately controlled by pitressin perfusions. PTEV, using Gelfoam soaked in sodium tetradecyl sulfate, controlled acute variceal bleeding in 71–95% of patients and appears to be more effective as an embolizing agent than bucrylate, which controlled 43–57%.

Considering the poor condition of the patients particularly during acute bleeding episodes, PTEV is a relatively safe therapeutic procedure that buys time for the surgeons to perform a decompressive shunt electively as definitive surgery. A one-year recurrent bleeding rate of 30% and a two year recurrence of 37.5% was noted. Thus, for long term control of variceal bleeding, a surgical decompressive shunt is recommended in addition to PTEV.

Key words: Gelfoam – Embolism, therapeutic – Catheters and catheterization – Esophagus, hemorrhage – Interventional radiology.

The technique of percutaneous transhepatic selective splanchnic vein cannulation via the right midaxillary approach was developed by Wiechel [25, 26]. Lunderquist [8] applied this technique to the occlusion of bleeding esophageal varices and in 1974 introduced this therapeutic modality into the United States, where it has been evaluated at several medical centers [5, 14, 20].

Address reprint requests to: W.C. Widrich, M.D., Department of Radiology, Boston Veterans Administration Hospital Center, 150 S. Huntington Ave., Jamaica Plain, MA 02130, USA

Evaluation and Initial Treatment of Patients

The variceal bleeding in the great majority of patients at the Boston Veterans Administration Medical Center is secondary to portal hypertension caused by alcoholic cirrhosis. Other, less common, causes are posthepatitic cirrhosis, postnecrotic cirrhosis, biliary cirrhosis, and extrahepatic portal hypertension.

Patients suspected of having esophagogastric variceal bleeding should be evaluated in the intensive care unit to determine the site of hemorrhage. Endoscopy has proved valuable in confirming the variceal bleeding and excluding other bleeding sites in the upper gastrointestinal tract. Even in patients with previously documented esophageal varices, endoscopy has shown that upper gastrointestinal bleeding occurs from other sites in 26–72% of cases [4, 12, 18]. If the bleeding source cannot be confirmed by endoscopy, or if a hepatoma or portal vein thrombosis is suspected, arteriography should be performed before transhepatic portography is attempted.

Many patients with cirrhosis and variceal bleeding have some sort of coagulopathy, defined as a prothrombin time greater than five seconds above control, a partial thromboplastin time greater than 15 seconds above control, or a platelet count of less than 50,000/mm^3. An inability to correct the coagulopathy resulted in poor control of bleeding by pitressin in six of 22 patients (27%) [10] and by PTEV in four of 16 (25%). Therefore, it is important that coagulation factor deficits be diagnosed quickly and the deficient factors be replaced aggressively.

We begin our attempts to control the variceal hemorrhage with a percutaneous intravenous infusion of pitressin at a rate of 0.4 units per minute [11, 13]. If the bleeding stops within the first four to six hours, the pitressin infusion is then tapered to a rate of 0.2 units per minute for 24 hours, then 0.1 units per minute for another 24 hours, and then discontinued. Patients whose bleeding is not adequately controlled with pitressin should have percutaneous transhepatic embolization of varices (PTEV) performed on an urgent basis.

Trauma to the mucosa overlying the varices, which can occur from gastritis, reflux esophagitis, or vomiting, may be the cause of the bleeding; mucosal healing is encouraged by the administration of cimetidine and antacids through the nasogastric tube.

PTEV Technique

Medication

Our patients are premedicated by the intramuscular administration of 75 mg of meperidine hydrochloride (Demerol) and 100 mg of sodium pentobarbital (Nembutal). These doses are modified in patients who are small, elderly, or in shock. The puncture site is infiltrated with 0.5% bupivocaine hydrochloride (Marcaine), which is a longer acting local anesthetic than lidocaine. Just before the first pass, a bolus of 6–12 mg of alphaprodine hydrochloride (Nisentil), a short acting narcotic, is injected intravenously; since its effect lasts for only a few minutes, the dose can be repeated once or twice without causing deep somnolence. This combination of medications has kept the vast majority of patients comfortable throughout the transhepatic procedure.

Technical Problems

In the transhepatic cannulation of the splanchnic veins [8, 19, 22], two technical problems may be encountered: (1) a densely fibrotic liver, which makes catheter advancement difficult, and (2) moderate to massive ascites, which increases the distance between the lateral abdominal wall and the liver. The catheter and guidewire tend to form a loop interfering with the selective catheterization of the desired venous branch. Both these problems can be overcome once the stiff part of an 0.035 inch floppy-tipped guide wire is well seated in the splenic or superior mesenteric vein. The catheter is removed and a stiff 5 French polyurethane introducer sheath[1] is advanced over the guide wire as far as it will go into the liver. The dilator is removed, leaving the sheath and guide wire in place. The 5 French catheter is then reinserted over the guide wire and through the sheath. Thus, friction from the liver is markedly reduced, and the sheath provides a firm support for the catheter across

the gap between the liver and the lateral abdominal wall. This maneuver also allows the catheter to be easily exchanged for a longer catheter or for reshaping.

When performing selective catheterizations, a 5 French Teflon sleeve is somewhat stiff and may not easily follow the guidewire into a selected vein. A polyethylene catheter[2] is softer and tends to follow the guide wire more readily. Also, curves can be steam-shaped easily on the tip of this catheter.

If the patient's coagulopathy is too severe for safe performance of the percutaneous transhepatic approach, one can gain access to the portal vein from the jugular vein. In this technique an 8 French Teflon catheter is introduced percutaneously into the right internal jugular vein and is passed through the right atrium into either the right or intermediate hepatic vein. A long, curved transeptal needle is advanced through the catheter until its sharp tip protrudes. The needle-catheter combination is advanced 2–3 cm into the liver, and the needle is removed. If the catheter tip is in the portal vein, the catheter can then be advanced over a guidewire to the desired position [6]. Another alternative is to pass a 5 French polyethylene catheter through the Teflon catheter for selective cannulation [24]. The advantage of the transjugular technique is that as the catheter is withdrawn, the patient bleeds into his own vascular system. The main disadvantage of this approach is the awkwardness of controlling the catheter as it is advanced through the liver.

Embolization Technique

Pressures are measured in the portal system and, if possible, compared to pressure measurements in the inferior vena cava.

A selective splenic venogram is performed to determine the position and number of all left gastric (coronary) and short gastric veins supplying the gastroesophageal varices. To control active bleeding, all veins supplying the varices must be occluded because most of these branches interconnect with one another. When the catheter is positioned well into the left gastric vein, the pitressin infusion is stopped, the balloons on the Sengstaken-Blakemore tube are deflated, and a selective left gastric venogram is performed.

Performance of a selective left gastric venogram before embolization is important. Spontaneous shunts between the left gastric vein directly entering the inferior vena cava, which occurred in 3% of the patients, might have resulted in emboli going directly to the

---

[1]   Cordis, Miami, Florida, USA

[2]   Hanafee, Becton-Dickinson Corporation, Rutherford, New Jersey 07070, USA

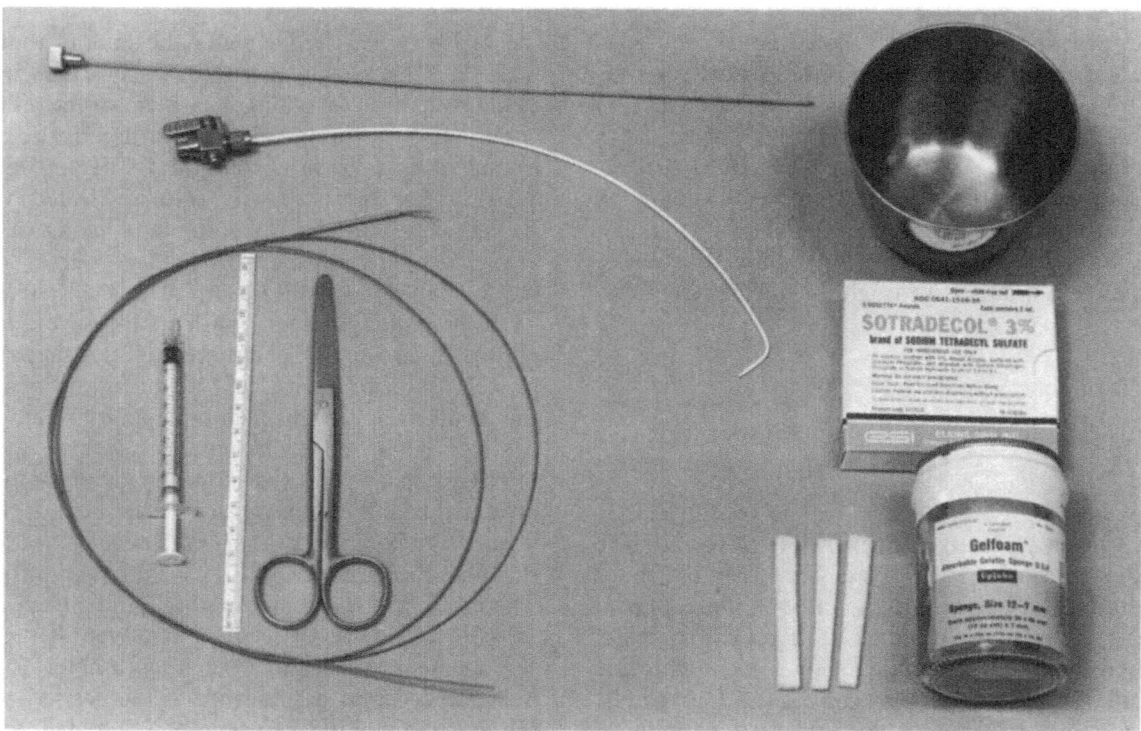

Fig. 1. Equipment for percutaneous transhepatic embolization of varices.

pulmonary arteries had these materials been injected. Additional venous communications from the left gastric vein to the left portal vein along the lesser curvature of the stomach occurred in 5% of the patients; emboli inadvertently entering the portal vein via this type of communication could be a potential complication [21].

PTEV is usually contraindicated in patients who have had a splenic vein occlusion or a thrombosed Warren-type distal selective splenorenal shunt. Blood in the left gastric vein in these patients was found to flow back toward the liver because the pressure in the splenic venous system markedly exceeded the pressure in the portal vein [21]. In such a situation injection of emboli into the left gastric vein would result in embolization of the portal vein. Splenectomy, or possibly the construction of an alternative portosystemic shunt, may be necessary to prevent recurrent variceal bleeding in such cases.

Before embolizing the varices, the catheter is positioned as selectively and as deeply as possible. Gelfoam strips are cut into 5-cm-long strips and soaked in 3% sodium tetradecyl sulfate (Sotradecol), a sclerosing agent used for thrombosing varicose veins in the leg (Fig. 1). One or two strips are loaded into the barrel of a 1-ml tuberculin syringe, the piston is reinserted, and the excess fluid is squeezed out. The mechanical advantage of the plastic tuberculin syringe can be best utilized if the volume of the squeezed contents is 0.5 ml or less. Just before embolization a test injection of contrast under fluoroscopic control will determine that the catheter tip has not changed position. The Gelfoam is steadily and firmly injected into the catheter. Again using the tuberculin syringe, contrast material in 0.5-ml increments is firmly injected to advance the Gelfoam along the catheter lumen. When the resistance of the Gelfoam begins to decrease, the injection force is eased. Under fluoroscopic control, the contrast material is gently injected until the Gelfoam is free of the catheter. This procedure is repeated until the vein is adequately occluded. As the catheter is removed from the occluded branch, 0.5 ml of contrast material is gently injected to prevent the catheter tip from dragging some of the Gelfoam into the splenic or portal vein.

After all the tributaries to the varices are occluded, a follow-up splenic venogram should be performed. Frequently, additional short gastric veins will opacify that will require embolization as well.

Embolic Materials

A variety of materials have been utilized to occlude varices. Powdered Gelfoam alternated with autologous heat-treated clot gave only temporary pro-

Table. Review of efficacy of transhepatic embolization of varices

	Number of patients	Material embolized	Control of active bleeding	Recurrent bleeding	Survival
Lunderquist et al. [9]	21	Isobutyl 2-cyanoacrylate	12/21 (57%) (1 month)		
Bengmark et al. [1]	43 14 active bleeders 30 elective	Isobutyl 2-cyano-acrylate	6/14 (43%) (1 month) (acute bleeders)	35% (1 week to 12 months)	26% at 34 months
Funaro et al. [5]	7	Gelfoam and stainless steel coils	1/7 (14%) (1 month)		
Viamonte et al. [17]	32	Gelfoam particles suspended in sodium tetradecyl sulfate	30/32 (94%)		
Pereiras et al. [15]	150	Gelfoam particles suspended in sodium tetradecyl sulfate	95% of 142 patients	30% (one year)	
Widrich et al. [23]	60 38 active bleeders	Gelfoam strips soaked in sodium tetradecyl sulfate	27/38 (71%) (1 month)		19/38 (50%) active bleeders (1 month)
	22 elective		20/22 (91%) (1 month)	37.5% at 2 years	12/22 (55%) elective patients (6 months to 4 years)

tection from variceal bleeding. Follow-up studies performed two months later showed that the previously occluded veins were totally patent [20]. Fogarty balloon occlusions of the left gastric vein also resulted in early recanalization. The balloons frequently leaked and became dislodged [20].

A combination of Gelfoam, thrombin, and etolein was used by Lunderquist et al. in their initial reports [7, 8]. Eight of 16 patients who underwent elective occlusion using this combination of materials had recurrent bleeding within 50 days of the procedure. Thirteen of 16 patients restudied had recanalization of the previously occluded veins five days to eight months later.

Lunderquist et al. subsequently employed isobutyl 2-cyanoacrylate (Bucrylate) [1, 9]. With this agent, bleeding was controlled for at least one week in eight of 14 (57%) actively bleeding patients whose bleeding was not controlled by the Sengstaken-Blakemore tube or by pitressin infusion (Table). Of 30 patients embolized electively, 11 (37%) had recurrent bleeding, mostly within one year of treatment.

Of seven patients who underwent transhepatic embolization of Gelfoam and stainless steel coils into the left gastric vein, six had recurrent bleeding within one month [5].

The combination of Gelfoam soaked in sodium tetradecyl sulfate seems to be the most reliable occluding agent in our experience [14, 20, 23]. The Gelfoam is caught in the interstices of the esophageal varices so that the sodium tetradecyl sulfate has prolonged contact with the intima of the veins resulting in a localized inflammatory response and usually long-term occlusion. Recanalization occurred in two of 23 patients up to two years after embolization [15].

Results

Control of Acute Variceal Bleeding

Pitressin infusion will initially control variceal bleeding in 80% of patients with portal hypertension; however, rebleeding will occur as the pitressin dosage is tapered off or after it is discontinued, so that complete control (for 30 days) is achieved in only 53% of the patients [10].

Control of acute variceal bleeding by PTEV was achieved in 94% [17] and 95% [15] of patients in two studies when Gelfoam particles suspended in sodium tetradecyl sulfate were used as the embolic agent. In patients whose bleeding was inadequately controlled by vasopressin (92% of whom were Child's Class C Category), a one-month control rate of 71% resulted when Gelfoam strips soaked in sodium tetradecyl sulfate were used [2, 23]. Bucrylate embolizations controlled 43–57% of active bleeders (30% of whom were Child's Class C Category) for one month [1, 9], while with Gelfoam and stainless steel coils, only one of seven patients (14%) was controlled for one month [5].

Protection from Additional Bleeding Episodes

Widrich et al. also performed elective PTEV as the definitive therapy in patients who had not bled for several days or weeks who were in one of several categories. These patients either (1) refused shunt surgery, (2) were those for whom the operative risks were prohibitive, (3) had prophylactic coronary vein occlusion before selective splenorenal shunt procedures, or (4) had PTEV as completion of surgical treatment, which had not involved ligation of the coronary vein. Using the life-table method, the recurrent bleeding rate at two years was 37.5% [23].

Pereiras et al. had a 30% one-year recurrent bleeding rate [15], while Bengmark et al. had a 35% recurrent bleeding rate at one week to 12 months [1].

Survival

Widrich et al. reported that 50% of active bleeders survived one month [23]. Ninety-two per cent were Child's Class C Category patients, and all were inadequately controlled with pitressin perfusions. Before the advent of PTEV, patients bleeding from esophageal varices, whether their bleeding was controlled by pitressin or not, had an in-hospital (one month) survival rate of 29–33% [3, 10]. Thus, in the active bleeders, PTEV appears to result in an increase in survival. In 12 of 22 patients (55%), elective PTEV was associated with a six month to four year survival [23]. Bengmark et al. found a 26% survival at the end of 34 months using life-table analysis [1].

Complications

The two most serious types of complications of PTEV are portal vein thrombosis and significant bleeding into the peritoneum from the puncture site.

Portal vein thrombosis is a common occurrence (21%) in patients with cirrhosis and is frequently associated with a fatal outcome (56% mortality) [16]. Six of the 43 (14%) active bleeders in Bengmark's report died within two months with associated portal vein thrombosis. Widrich et al. noted five complications of portal vein thrombosis (two fatal) in 60 patients (8%) [23]. Three of the five were incidental findings noted at angiography; these three patients had no clinical symptoms or hepatic chemistry changes.

Significant bleeding into the peritoneum in two (one fatal) of 60 patients (3%) was reported by Widrich et al. and in three (one fatal) of 43 patients (7%) by Bengmark et al. Bleeding of this sort can be reduced by insertion of a Gelfoam plug into the liver puncture site as the catheter is removed.

Pleural effusion requiring a chest tube occurred in one of 60 patients in Widrich's series and in one of 43% patients in Bengmark's series.

Less serious complications included fever, ascitic leak, and clinically insignificant subcapsular hematomas [15, 23].

References

1. Bengmark, S., Börjesson, B., Hoevels, J., Joelsson, B., Lunderquist, A., Owman, T.: Obliteration of esophageal varices by PTP. Ann. Surg. 190:549–554, 1979
2. Child, C.G., III: The Liver and Portal Hypertension. Philadelphia, Saunders, 1964
3. Conn, H.O.: The prognosis and managment of bleeding esophageal varices. Ann. N.Y. Acad. Sci. 170:345, 1970
4. Dagradi, A., Mehler, R., Tan, D., Stempien, S.: Sources of upper gastrointestinal bleeding in patients with liver cirrhosis and large esophagogastric varices. Am. J. Gastroenterol. 54:458–463, 1970
5. Funaro, A., Ring, E.J., Freiman, D.B., Oleaga, J., Gordon, R.L.: Transhepatic obliteration of esophageal varices using the stainless steel coil. Am. J. Roentgenol. 133:1123–1125, 1979
6. Goldman, M.L., Fajman, W., Galambos, J.: Transjugular obliteration of the gastric coronary vein. Radiology 118:453–455, 1976
7. Lunderquist, A., Simert, G., Tylen, U., Vang, J.: Follow-up of patients with portal hypertension and esophageal varices treated with percutaneous obliteration of gastric coronary vein. Radiology 122:59–63, 1977
8. Lunderquist, A., Vang, J.: Transhepatic catheterization and obliteration of the coronary vein in patients with portal hypertension and esophageal varices. N. Engl. J. Med. 291:646–649, 1974
9. Lunderquist, A., Borjesson, B., Owman, T., Bengmark, S.: Isobutyl 2-cyanoacrylate (Bucrylate) in obliteration of gastric coronary vein and esophageal varices. Am. J. Roentgenol. 130:1–6, 1978

10. Johnson, W.C., Widrich, W.C.: Efficacy of selective splanchnic arteriography and vasopressin perfusion in the diagnosis and treatment of gastrointestinal hemorrhage. Am. J. Surg. 131:481–489, 1976

11. Johnson, W.C., Widrich, W.C., Ansell, J., Robbins, A.H., Nabseth, D.C.: Control of bleeding varices by vasopressin: A prospective randomized study. Ann. Surg. 186:369–376, 1977

12. McCray, R.S., Martin, F., Amir-Ahmadi, H., Sheahan, D.G., Zamcheck, N.: Erroneous diagnosis of hemorrhage from esophageal varices. Am. J. Dig. Dis. 14:755–760, 1969

13. Nusbaum M., Baum, S., Kuroda, K., Blakemore, W.S.: Control of portal hypertension by selective mesenteric arterial infusion. Arch. Surg. 97:1005–1013, 1968

14. Pereiras, R., Viamonte, M., Russell, E., LePage, J., White, P., Hutson, D.: New techniques for interruption of gastroesophageal venous blood flow. Radiology 124:313–323, 1977

15. Pereiras, R., Schiff, E., Barkin, J., Hutson, D.: The role of interventional radiology in diseases of the hepatobiliary system and the pancreas. Radiol. Clin. North Am. 17:555–605, 1979

16. Sarfeh, I.J.: Portal vein thrombosis associated with cirrhosis. Arch. Surg. 114:902–905, 1979

17. Viamonte, M., Pereiras, R., Russell, E., LePage, J., Hutson, D.: Transhepatic obliteration of gastroesophageal varices: Results in acute and nonacute bleeders. Am. J. Roentgenol. 129:237–241, 1977

18. Waldram, R., Davis, M., Nunnerley, H., Williams, R.: Emergency endoscopy after gastrointestinal hemorrhage in 50 patients with portal hypertension. Br. Med. J. 4:94–96, 1974

19. Widrich, W.C., Robbins, A.H., Nabseth, D.C., O'Hara, E.T., Johnson, W.C., Laughlin, K.V.: Portal hypertension changes following selective splenorenal shunt surgery. Radiology 121:295–302, 1976

20. Widrich, W.C., Johnson, W.C., Robbins, A.H., Nabseth, D.C.: Esophagogastric variceal hemorrhage. Arch. Surg. 113:1331–1338, 1978

21. Widrich, W.C., Robbins, A.H., Nabseth, D.C., Johnson, W.C., Goldstein, S.A.: Pitfalls of transhepatic portal venography and therapeutic coronary vein occlusion. Am. J. Roentgenol. 131:637–643, 1978

22. Widrich, W.C., Robbins, A.H., Johnson, W.C., Nabseth, D.C.: Long-term follow-up of distal splenorenal shunts. Radiology 134:341–345, 1980

23. Widrich, W.C., Johnson, W.C., Robbins, A.H., Nabseth, D.C.: Transhepatic Variceal Occlusion. New York, Academic Press (in press)

24. Widrich, W.C., Sequeira, S.R.: Interventional radiology of the liver and related structures. Radiol. Clin. North Am. (in press)

25. Wiechel, K.L.: Percutaneous transhepatic cholangiography. Acta Chir. Scand. (Suppl.) 330:1–99, 1964

26. Wiechel, K.L.: Tekniken vid perkutan transhepatisk portapunkton (PTP) (abstr.). Nord. Med. 86:912, 1971

Comment

Transhepatic Embolization of Varices: A Surgeon's View

Ronald A. Malt

Department of Surgery, Harvard Medical School, and Surgical Services, Massachusetts General Hospital, Boston, Massachusetts, USA

Anthropologists interested in the effect of geography on genetic diversity should ignore the subleties introduced by continental drift and concentrate instead on the enormous differences across the few miles that separate our hospital from the Boston Veterans Administration Hospital. Whereas across town variceal bleeding can be acutely controlled for one month in 71% of patients, resulting in a 51% mortality rate at the end of that time, the results of PTEV are much worse on the banks of the Charles – or, for that matter, in midtown Philadelphia. Here, only five of 19 patients (22%) had their variceal bleeding controlled for the duration of their hospital stay; all who rebled were in Child's class C and died (78% overall mortality rate) [1]. At the Hospital of the University of Pennsylvania (E. Ring, unpublished data), bleeding

Address reprint requests to: R.A. Malt, M.D., Surgical Services, Massachusetts General Hospital, Fruit Street, Boston, MA 02114, USA

was controlled in none of 18 class C patients, and all 18 died.

How can one resolve the disparity between the results of a procedure that has been endorsed by Widrich and his colleagues, but has been followed by such high lethality in two other institutions that it has been abandoned completely? The most obvious explanation would be that our vascular radiologists (and those at Pennsylvania) do not know how to obliterate varices properly. In view of the feats of legerdemain habitually performed by my collaborators in the angiography department, I reject this hypothesis.

Second would be the possibility that the ostensibly good results are interpreted too enthusiastically. This hypothesis I reject, too, since Dr. Nabseth is a supreme skeptic about data presented by either fellow surgeons or radiological associates [2].

Results of every kind of treatment for cirrhotic patients depend largely on the hepatic reserve of the patients [3–5]. For example, after transthoracic ligation of esophageal varices at our hospital, about 100% of class A patients survive, as do 55% of class B and 10% of class C [6]. Therefore, given approximately equal methods of treatment and even-handedness in assessing outcomes, there must be differences in the ways the various hospitals are classifying their patients according to hepatic function.

Unless PTEV is qualitatively different from any other form of therapy, I suspect that in a randomized and stratified trial, results of PTEV would be equivalent among all hospitals. Although Child's [7] stratification of cirrhotic patients was a great stroke of induction, which has proved widely useful as a first approximation, few physicians when questioned actually seem to know the five criteria defining it; those who do, rarely use all five. Moreover, how can a patient be precisely categorized if, for example, his serum bilirubin level is 1.9 mg/dl (pointing toward category A), while his albumin level is 2.8 g/dl (pointing toward category C)? When authors state that most of their patients are category C, but can have their coagulopathy corrected rapidly by administration of exogenous clotting factors, I wonder if their *C* is our *C*. Because the livers of our C-risk patients are rotten, no treatment corrects their coagulation defects for more than an equilibration time.

Since both our studies [4, 5] and those of Orloff and associates [8,9] sharpen the discriminants of hepatic function, it would seem preferable to adopt a deductively derived, reliable, sensitive, and linear means of assessment. The one we support for prediction of results after splenorenal or portacaval shunting is based on a table essayable from the last liver function tests determined before operation (Table) [4].

Table. Scale for predicting operative mortality

Predictor	Points assigned		
	0	1	2
Bilirubin (mg/dl)	≦0.99	1.00–1.99	≧2.0
Ascites	None	Controlled (stable)	Uncontrollable
Operative urgency	Elective	Emergency	–

Score is the sum of points assigned for each predictor: minimum =0, maximum=5.

A score of 0 predicts a 0% mortality rate, 2 predicts approximately 10%, 3 predicts 40%, 4 predicts 60%, and 5 predicts nearly 100% mortality rate.

Finally, I wonder whether PTEV has been validated in an animal model having high-pressure distensible veins. I never consider Gelfoam useful for any purpose in vascular surgery, and I expect that sodium tetradecyl sulfate (Sotradecol) would be rapidly cleared from a vein. When sodium tetradecyl sulfate injection is chosen for treatment of varicose veins of the lower extremity, obliteration does not occur unless the vein walls are compressed for a few days, or preferably, a few weeks. When angiography was performed here on one B-risk patient shortly after PTEV done elsewhere, the coronary veins and varices were patent. Even when varices are totally obliterated with isobutyl 2-cyanoacrylate [10] many patients still bleed.

References

1. Athanasoulis, C.A.: Therapeutic applications of angiography. N. Engl. J. Med. 302:1117–1125 and 1174–1179, 1980
2. Malt, R.A., Nabseth, D.C., Orloff, M.J., Stipa, S.: Portal hypertension, 1979. N. Engl. J. Med. 301:617–618, 1979
3. Malt, R.A.: Portasystemic venous shunts. N. Engl. J. Med. 295:24–29 and 80–86, 1976
4. Malt, R.A., Szczerban, J., Malt, R.B.: Risks in therepeutic portacaval and splenorenal shunts. Ann. Surg. 184:279–288, 1976
5. Malt, R.B., Malt, R.A.: Tests and mangement affecting survival after portacaval and splenorenal shunts. Surg. Gynecol. Obstet. 149:220–224, 1979
6. Ottinger, L.W., Moncure, A.C.: Transthoracic ligation of bleeding esophageal varices in patients with portal obstruction. Ann. Surg. 179:35, 1977
7. Child, C.G., III, Turcotte, J.G.: Surgery and portal hypertension. In: The Liver and Portal Hypertension, edited by C.G. Child, III. Philadelphia, W.B. Saunders, 1964, pp. 1–85
8. Orloff, M.J., Charters, A.C., III, Chandler, J.G., Condon, J.K., Grambort, D.E., Modafferi, T.R., Levin, S.E., Brown, N.B., Sviokla, S.C., Knox, D.G.: Portacaval shunt as an emergency procedure in unselected patients with alcoholic cirrhosis. Surg. Gynecol. Obstet. 141:59–68, 1975
9. Orloff, M.J., Bell, R.H., Jr, Hyde, P.V., et al.: Long-term results of emergency portacaval shunt for bleeding esophageal varices in unselected patients with alcoholic cirrhosis. Ann. Surg. (in press)
10. Bengmark, S., Börjesson, B., Hoevels, J., Joelsson, B., Lunderquist, A., Owman, T.: Obliteration of esophageal varices by PTP: A follow-up of 43 patients. Ann. Surg. 190:549–554, 1979

Reply

Warren C. Widrich, Alan H. Robbins, and Donald C. Nabseth

We would like to thank Dr. Malt for his picturesque and interesting comments.

The angiographic abilities of our colleagues on the same bank of the Charles River and in midtown Philadelphia are, indeed, superb. A meaningful comparison between our experience and any other experience with PTEV, however, can be made only if the same method is used, with the same embolic materials, in approximately the same type of patients. The question to ask the MGH, Ring et al., and Bengmark et al. is: What has been your experience with patient survival and arrest of esophageal hemorrhage for 30 days in alcoholic patients in whom bleeding was not controlled by other means, using PTEV with Gelfoam strips soaked in sodium tetradecyl sulfate?

PTEV controlled variceal bleeding in a significant number of our patients whose bleeding was not controlled by pitressin infusions or other conservative means. One difference between our experience and others is our use of Gelfoam strips soaked in sodium tetradecyl sulfate. Except for one case, the previously embolized veins in over 17 of our patients were still occluded on follow-up transhepatic portal venograms up to 11 months later. As is stated in the manuscript, Pereiras performed embolization using Gelfoam soaked in sodium tetradecyl sulfate and controlled acutely bleeding varices in 95% of his patients; recanalization occurred in two of 23 patients followed up to two years after embolization.

Another difference may be that we have an enthusiastic hematology team that is involved in the care of these patients early on and will aggressively replace deficient coagulation factors. Correction of these coagulopathies has been an important factor in determining success or failure to control bleeding. Despite this help, 13 of the 38 actively bleeding patients in our series had significant coagulopathy (as defined in our paper) at the time of PTEV.

Child's classification was designed to predict the survival of patients undergoing a portacaval shunt. There is some variation from clinician to clinician

in interpreting the five factors involved in the Child's classification. Orloff and associates, in a recent report at the American Surgical Association (April 1980), found in a consecutive series of 181 patients subjected to portacaval shunt that traditionally invoked risk factors that had no significant influence on survival included age, jaundice, encephalopathy, muscle wasting, delirium tremens, a small liver, and results of the usual liver function tests such as serum bilirubin and albumin levels.

Be that as it may, in our series of 38 actively bleeding patients, control of bleeding (i.e., requiring no more than two units of blood transfusion within one month after PTEV) and one-month survival were as follows:

Child's classification	No. of patients	Control of bleeding	One-month survival
A	2 (5%)	2/2 (100%)	2/2 (100%)
B	2 (5%)	1/2 (50%)	2/2 (100%)
C	34 (90%)	24/34 (71%)	15/34 (44%)
Total	38 (100%)	27/38 (71%)	19/38 (50%)

We then categorized our patients according to Dr. Malt's classification. Urgency of PTEV was substituted for operative urgency:

Malt's classification	No. of patients	Control of bleeding	One-month survival
0	0 (0%)	—	—
1	1 (3%)	1/1 (100%)	1/1 (100%)
2	3 (8%)	2/3 (67%)	3/3 (100%)
3	7 (18%)	4/7 (57%)	4/7 (57%)
4	17 (45%)	13/17 (76%)	11/17 (65%)
5	10 (26%)	7/10 (70%)	0/10 (0%)
Total	38 (100%)	27/38 (71%)	19/38 (50%)

Reply

Ronald A. Malt

Category 5 patients are the very ones with whom we have the most trouble. They are the ones who do not stop bleeding spontaneously and the ones whose coagulation defects we cannot correct. They are the ones whose bleeding is refractory to balloon tamponade, to vasopressin, to most attempts at surgery, and, apparently, to PTEV. *Res ipse loquitur,* I guess.

Final Remarks

Control of Bleeding Esophageal Varices by Endoscopic Sclerotherapy

W. Rösch

Department of Medicine, University of Erlangen-Nürnberg, Erlangen, FRG

Suitable therapy of bleeding esophageal varices has been a challenge for the gastroenterologist for many years. Despite many attempts no generally accepted breakthrough has been achieved, although several new methods such as transhepatic embolization are promising. In West Germany a different approach is currently favored and practiced in most institutions: injection therapy, introduced in 1939 by Crafoord and Frenckner [1], has been broadly accepted by endoscopists as it combines diagnostic and therapeutic measures. The results of Terblanche et al. [3] gained in a prospective evaluation are convincing: hemorrhage was controlled in 92% with a mortality rate of 25%. Although similar success (91.3%) was reported by Kiefhaber et al. [2] using the neodymium YAG laser for hemostasis in bleeding varices, recurrent hemorrhage in 28 of 127 patients required intermittent sclerosing or shunt procedures. Paquet [2] using the rigid esophagoscope for sclerosing recently published long-term data on 858 patients who were treated between 1969 and 1979. Of these patients 66.5% are alive, 13.5% died in hospital, 14% died at home, and 6% were not available for follow-up. In contrast to most authors Soehendra [2] uses a flexible endoscope and injects the sclerosing agent directly into the varices. Hemorrhage was controlled in 92.6%, and the mortality rate was 24% within the first year. Sclerosing is also beginning to be used prophylactically.

The following questions still remain unresolved: (1) whether a rigid esophagoscope is superior in sclerosing to a flexible instrument, (2) whether paravasal injection gives better long-term results than intravasal instillation, and (3) whether sclerosing at regular intervals is superior to shunt procedures after successful endoscopic arrest of hemorrhage. However, it must be mentioned that Denck and Olbert [2] combine sclerosing technique with transhepatic embolization in hemorrhage of fundic varices. It is our opinion that sclerosing of bleeding varices is a rational approach during urgent endoscopy and that temporary arrest can be achieved in almost all patients. Further measures depend primarily on liver function, and in patients suitable for elective shunt operations we consider surgical decompression preferable.

References

1. Crafoord, C., Frenckner, P.: New surgical treatment of varicose veins of the oesophagus. Acta Otolaryngol. (Stockh.) 27:422–429 (1939)
2. Demling, L., Rösch, W.: Operative Endoskopie 1979. Acron, Berlin 1979
3. Terblanche, J., Northover, J.M.A., Bornman, P., Kahn, D., Barbezat, G.O., Sellars, S.L., Saunders, S.J.: A prospective evaluation of injection sclerotherapy in the treatment of acute bleeding from esophageal varices. Surgery 85:239–245 (1979)

Address reprint requests to: Prof. Dr. W. Rösch, Medizinische Klinik mit Poliklinik der Universität Erlangen-Nürnberg, Krankenhausstr. 12, D-8520 Erlangen, Federal Republic of Germany

Transvenous Devices
for the Management of Pulmonary Embolism

Morris Simon, and Aubrey M. Palestrant

Department of Radiology, Harvard Medical School and Beth Israel Hospital, Boston, Massachusetts, USA

Abstract. When anticoagulant treatment of pulmonary embolism is contraindicated or fails, interruption of blood flow through the inferior vena cava offers an alternative method for preventing further embolic episodes. In the past this required abdominal surgery, but currently several clot-capturing devices have been designed for insertion into the human inferior vena cava indirectly via a jugular or femoral venotomy. Another device is being developed for percutaneous delivery through a standard angiographic catheter. In addition to variations in the delivery methods, the form, mechanical effectiveness, and complications of these differ markedly. A suction-cup device is also available for the transvenous removal of pulmonary emboli.

Key words: Embolism, pulmonary – Vena cava, transvenous interruption – Interventional radiology.

While evidence of pulmonary embolism is commonly found in routine autopsies [1], most patients survive the embolic episodes so that the true incidence of pulmonary embolism is difficult to determine [2]. It has been estimated that in the United States there will be about 630,000 cases of significant pulmonary embolism this year. In hospitalized patients, it is a common cause of morbidity and mortality, accounting for approximately 200,000 deaths in the United States each year [3]. Symptoms ensue only when the embolus is large, and only those greater than 7.5 mm in diameter are likely to be fatal, although preexisting cardiopulmonary disease increases a patient's vulnerability [4]. Some patients sustain a pulmonary embolism as the final episode of a terminal illness, but

Address reprint requests to: M. Simon, M.D., Department of Radiology, Beth Israel Hospital, 330 Brookline Ave., Boston, MA 02115, USA

at least one-half of the fatal episodes occur in patients who would otherwise have a good prognosis. The incidence of recurrent pulmonary embolism is estimated at 60%, including a fatal recurrence rate of 22% without treatment [2]. Accurate diagnosis and early treatment is important and has been shown to increase patient survival greatly [5].

Indications for Inferior Vena Cava Interruption

Most patients with documented pulmonary embolism are treated effectively by anticoagulation. More recently, thrombolytic drugs have been used to accelerate the normal thrombolytic process in massive pulmonary embolism. In some patients, however, these methods of treatment are inappropriate. Since most pulmonary emboli originate from veins in the lower limbs, pelvis, or inferior vena cava, mechanical interruption of the inferior vena cava is then necessary to prevent a life-threatening pulmonary embolus from reaching the lungs.

Current indications for interrupting the inferior vena cava are:

1. Pulmonary embolism in patients with a high risk of internal bleeding, a contraindication to anticoagulant or thrombolytic therapy. Such patients include those who have had recent trauma, surgery, cerebral hemorrhage, or peptic ulcer disease.

2. Recurrent pulmonary embolism despite adequate anticoagulant therapy. While heparin prevents further thrombosis, it does not affect an already formed thrombus, nor does it prevent detachment of a previously propagated thrombus in a major vein. Thrombolysis of recent thrombi usually takes three to seven days, during which time all or part of the thrombus may embolize. Recurrent embolism therefore does not always represent a failure of anticoagulant therapy. In the first few days after initiation of therapy, ineffective anticoagulation associated with

continued thrombus formation can only be demonstrated by radioactive fibrinogen uptake studies or serial phlebography [4].

3. Phlebographic demonstration of potentially fatal thrombi in the iliofemoral veins or inferior vena cava. Patients with large free-floating thrombi are considered to be at great risk of developing fatal embolism [6].

4. As prophylaxis against pulmonary embolism in elderly patients with hip fractures or other high-risk conditions. Pulmonary embolism was the cause of death in 38% of patients who died following hip fractures [7]. In one study the prophylactic insertion of an inferior vena cava filter device in these patients reduced the incidence of clinically detectable emboli from 20% in the control group to 0% in the group with filters [8].

5. Pulmonary embolism associated with heparin sensitivity, which may cause disseminated thrombosis and profound thrombocytopenia in some patients [9]. Since no other anticoagulant drug acts as rapidly as heparin, inferior vena cava interruption is an alternative choice for early treatment.

6. Prevention of recurrent pulmonary embolism after pulmonary thrombolectomy [10].

Methods of Interrupting the Vena Cava

During the past 35 years a variety of approaches to the interruption of the inferior vena cava have been used in the treatment of pulmonary embolism. Originally these required abdominal surgery, but recently devices have been inserted via a jugular or femoral venotomy requiring surgical dissection remote from the vena cava.

Surgical Transabdominal Approaches

Initially a direct surgical approach was used. O'Neill first described ligation of the inferior vena cava for prevention of pulmonary embolism in 1945 [11]. However, the complete occlusion of the inferior vena cava is soon followed by enlargement of collateral channels, which can allow passage of potentially fatal emboli [12]. The search for an improved surgical approach focused upon techniques of partial occlusion of the vena cava. Suture filters [13], suture partitioning [14], bead compression [15], and external clips [16] (Fig. 1) have been used. However, these methods all required major abdominal surgery under general anesthesia, often in seriously ill patients. Anticoagulant therapy had to be suspended before, during, and after the operation, increasing the risk of further thrombus formation during this period. In a review

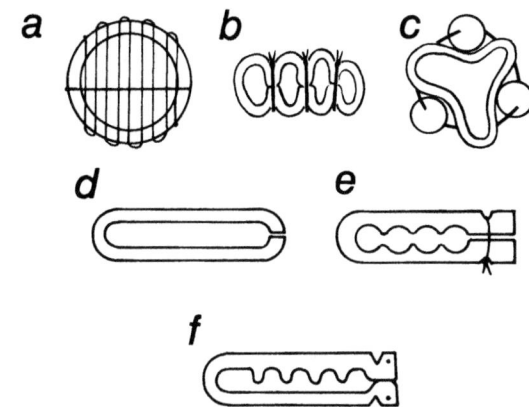

Fig. 1. Surgical techniques for inferior vena caval interruption. *a* DeWeese suture filter. *b* Spencer suture partition. *c* Mozes bead compression. *d* Moretz clip. *e* Miles clip. *f* Adams-DeWeese clip.

of a number of surgical series, the reported operative mortality was found to range from 0 to 39% with a mean of 9.9%, recurrent embolism from 0 to 30% with a mean of 5.96%, and fatal recurrences from 0 to 22% with a mean of 1.96% [17].

The most popular surgical method employed today is the placement of a fenestrated clip around the inferior vena cava [16]. This form of caval interruption is often performed as a prophylactic measure in the course of abdominal surgery for the patient's primary disease if there is a high risk of postoperative pulmonary thromboembolism [18]. At the same time, potentially large collateral channels such as the gonadal veins may also be interrupted. The patency rate of the fenestrated clip is 85% [19].

Transvenous Approaches

The indirect transvenous placement of an intraluminal device in the inferior vena cava is an attractive approach since it substitutes a minor surgical procedure, the dissection of a peripheral vein in the neck or groin, for major abdominal surgery. This method requires less operating time, has lower morbidity, and reduces the recuperation period. The same hemodynamic result is achieved at substantially reduced cost.

Development of Transvenous Devices

The transvenous devices first developed included the Eichelter sieve [20] and the Moser balloon [21] (Fig. 2). These were designed to provide temporary protection against embolism during the early, vulnerable period. In each case, the device remained at-

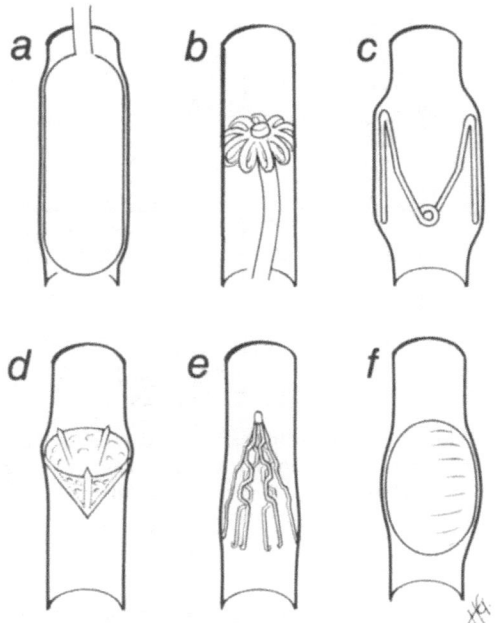

Fig. 2. Transvenous devices for inferior vena caval interruption. *a* Moser balloon. *b* Eichelter sieve. *c* Pate clip. *d* Mobin-Uddin umbrella filter. *e* Kimray-Greenfield filter. *f* Hunter balloon.

tached to a catheter with its proximal end outside the body. The catheter surface, vessel puncture site, and other sites of intimal injury were potential sources of thrombus formation, and captured emboli or newly formed thrombus could be released into the blood stream when the device was withdrawn. These devices were the subject of several experimental reports but were not used in humans.

A more effective transvenous approach was the delivery of a detachable device that served as a permanent barrier to emboli. Such devices acted in one of three ways: (1) by narrowing the vena cava into a slit-like cross section (Pate clip [22]), (2) by total occlusion of the lumen (Hunter balloon [23]), and (3) by filtering the blood flow (Mobin-Uddin umbrella [24] and Kimray-Greenfield filter [25]) (Fig. 3). The last three devices are in current clinical usage and will be described in greater detail.

Insertion of Transvenous Devices

Venacavography is usually performed to assess the patency and anatomy of the vena cava and the levels of the renal veins so that an optimal position for the device can be chosen. A left femoral vein approach is used since the chances of demonstrating inferior vena cava anomalies, such as a double inferior vena cava, are greater than if the procedure is done through the right femoral vein [26] (Fig. 4). An initial injection

of a small quantity of contrast medium is observed fluoroscopically to ensure that there is no thrombus at or above the puncture site. An angiographic catheter is then inserted by the standard Seldinger technique and venacavography is performed.

The techniques for inserting current transvenous devices are similar in many respects. The patient is sedated, and after local anesthesia an incision is made on the right side of the neck to expose the internal jugular vein by careful dissection. The device and its delivery apparatus are passed through a jugular venotomy and maneuvered through the right atrium of the heart and into the inferior vena cava under fluoroscopic control. The Hunter balloon and Kimray-Greenfield filter delivery systems allow injection of contrast through the catheter to check the position of the device prior to its release.

The optimal position for the device is just below the lowest renal vein so that the space between the device and the vein is as small as possible, since if the device were to become occluded by a large thrombus the stagnant blood in this space could thrombose and become a source of emboli. After insertion of the device, follow-up phlebography helps to demonstrate the position of the device in the vena cava and to determine if there have been any complications from the procedure, e.g., perforation, hemorrhage, or early thrombus formation on the filter. Capture of emboli during the course of the procedure has also been documented.

Patients should not be anticoagulated for 12 hours after a filter has been inserted because of the potential for hemorrhage at the sites of penetration by anchoring hooks or spokes. The importance of prophylactic antibiotic administration during and after the insertion of a device, as is current practice with prosthetic heart valves, remains an unresolved question. The use of prophylactic antibiotics may also be prudent when patients with these devices are at risk for bacteremia, e.g., after surgery or dental extraction. Bacteremia causing infection of a thrombosed umbrella filter has been described [27].

Transvenous Devices Currently in Use

Mobin-Uddin Umbrella Filter (Fig. 2). This filter was first described in 1967 [28] and its use in human subjects reported in 1969 [29]. Since then, several thousand have been successfully inserted. The filter is a miniature umbrella with six flat stainless steel spokes radiating from a central hub and covered by a thin Silastic membrane impregnated with heparin. The tips of the spokes are sharpened to perforate the caval wall in order to anchor the filter in place. There are

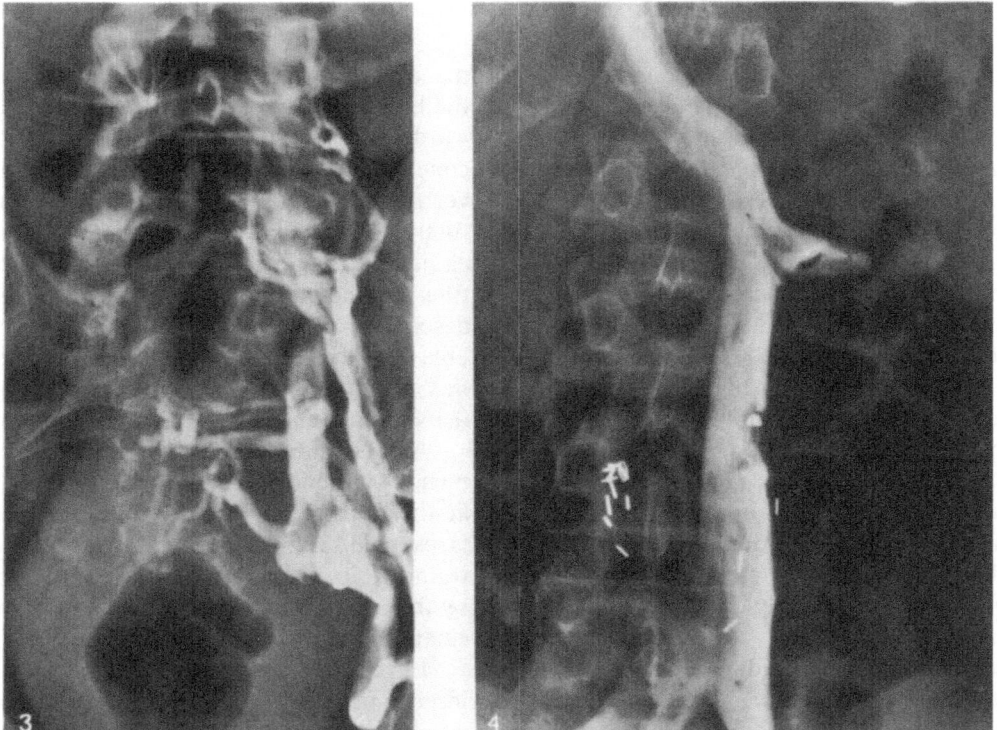

Fig. 3. Mobin-Uddin umbrella filter. A left femoral vein injection shows occlusion of the inferior vena cava and the development of collateral channels.

Fig. 4. Kimray-Greenfield filter. Left femoral vein injection. Note anomalous left-sided inferior vena cava containing a filter tilted to one side. Captured thrombus is demonstrated inside and outside the filter.

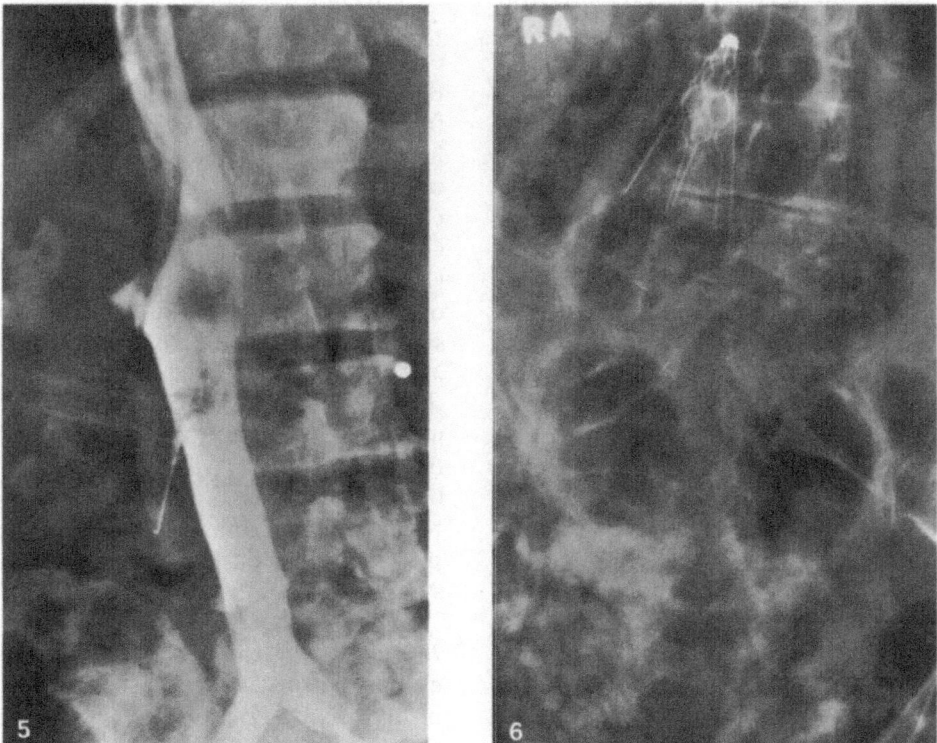

Fig. 5. Kimray-Greenfield filter. Device has perforated the inferior vena cava and lies tilted in the lumen. Note captured thrombus both within and outside the filter.

Fig. 6. Kimray-Greenfield filter. Right femoral vein injection. There is total occlusion of the inferior vena cava with diversion of contrast medium into pelvic and large gonadal veins, a potential route for large emboli.

115

eighteen 3 mm fenestrations in the Silastic membrane. Originally a 23 mm diameter filter was used, but episodes of filter migration led to the development of a larger 28 mm filter. The filter is folded into the delivery capsule with the spokes approximated. The delivery capsule measures 7 mm in diameter and 32 mm in length and is attached to a spiral wound guide wire through which the release core-wire slides. The filter is inserted into the inferior vena cava with its apex directed downward, using the technique outlined above. The filter springs open like an umbrella when released, an action that allows it to adapt to smaller inferior vena cavas.

Heparin therapy is withheld for 12 hours after insertion of the umbrella filter to minimize the possibility of retroperitoneal bleeding from the perforating spokes. Oral anticoagulants are started on the third postoperative day and are usually continued for three months or longer.

The umbrella insertion procedure is generally uneventful, but several complications have been reported. These include the accidental lodging of the device in the right renal vein, the right common iliac vein, and the suprarenal inferior vena cava; retroperitoneal hematoma; hemorrhage and air embolism from the venotomy site; right recurrent laryngeal nerve injury; thrombosis above the filter [30]; and perforation of the duodenum and right ureter [24]. Pressure gradients across the filter as high as 20 mm Hg have been reported. This may predispose to venostasis, edema, and thrombophlebitis in the lower limbs.

Recurrent embolism with the 28-mm filter has been reported in 0.5% of 2,562 placements [31]. The older 23-mm filter had an incidence of 3% recurrence, a quarter of which were fatal. The incidence of inferior vena caval occlusion with the newer heparin-bonded filter is 60% (Fig. 3). Leg edema occurred in 5.1% of patients and lower extremity phlebitis in 1.5%, but these conditions usually respond to standard medical treatment. Filter migration occurred in 0.4%. When the filter migrated proximally, nine of 22 patients died as a result of the acute episode or related surgery [24]. Distal migration has been documented following cardiac massage, presumably due to a water-hammer effect.

Kimray-Greenfield Filter (Fig. 2). The Kimray-Greenfield filter was first described in 1973 [32], and the initial clinical series was published in 1977 [25]. The device consists of six 0.015 inch tempered stainless steel wires extending from a small hub to form a cone with a maximal apical angle of 35 degrees. The wires measure 4.6 cm in length, and the tips form a circular base with a maximum diameter of 3.0 cm. Sharp hooks at the ends of the wire arms engage

the caval wall and prevent filter migration toward the heart. Since the apex of the filter is directed upward, its conical shape permits filling of 70% of the cone by blood clot with a decrease in the inferior vena cava's effective cross section by only 50%. The filter is loaded into a capsule that is attached to a catheter containing the release wire. Delivery of the filter to the inferior vena cava follows the outline described above. A modified delivery system is available for filter insertion through the femoral vein, but this route is associated with a greater incidence of delivery complications.

At the time of filter insertion, Greenfield recommends that blood coagulation times be maintained at the upper limits of normal. Full anticoagulation is resumed 12 hours after placement if there are no contraindications. Long-term anticoagulation is dictated by the underlying thrombotic disorder but is not necessary to maintain long-term patency of the filter [25].

Infrequent complications associated with the filter insertion include failure to pass the capsule into the inferior vena cava; misplacement into the right atrium or hepatic or renal veins; incorrect orientation, with the filter tilted to one or other side (Fig. 4); wound hematoma; and retroperitoneal hemorrhage. We have observed one filter perforation without symptoms (Fig. 5).

Greenfield reported his clinical experience with 76 patients, indicating that the inferior vena caval occlusion rate is low (3%) (Fig. 6). There have been no reported cases of proximal migration, although two filters migrated distally without ill effect [33]. The incidence of recurrent embolism, diagnosed on the basis of symptoms, is reported to be 2.6%. Other complications encountered after filter insertion include thrombophlebitis (5.2%) and extremity edema (11.8%). No deaths were related to filter insertion or malfunction. Thrombus has been observed on both sides of the filter in follow-up venograms (Figs. 4 and 5). In three of four patients in Greenfield's series, the thrombi were not apparent on subsequent examinations. Greenfield's explanation of this finding is that the thrombi are lysed in situ by the flow of blood around them. A further possibility is fragmentation of the thrombus into parts small enough to pass through the filter but too small to cause clinical symptoms when they reach the lungs.

Hunter Occlusion Balloon (Fig. 2). This balloon occlusion device, which was first described and used in humans by Hunter in 1970 [34], consists of a detachable ribbed balloon at the tip of a 75-cm-long delivery catheter with a needle inside the catheter connecting the balloon to an inflation syringe. Insertion of the delivery mechanism into the inferior vena cava follows the general method outlined previously, and contrast may be injected through the catheter to check its position in the inferior vena cava. The balloon is positioned below the renal veins and is inflated with contrast medium until it stretches the cava and cannot be moved by firm tugging on the catheter. The catheter is then detached, leaving the balloon in place. If blood clot is encountered in the inferior vena cava above the renal veins during the insertion procedure, the balloon may be partially inflated and used as a piston to push the clot below the renal veins. The balloon causes total occlusion of the distal cava and thus forces the blood to flow through collateral channels.

An advantage of the balloon method of caval interruption is that anticoagulation of the patient need not be suspended during and after the balloon insertion since there are no anchoring hooks or points to penetrate the vein wall. Half of Hunter's patients were anticoagulated during and after balloon placement without any reported complications, including retroperitoneal hemorrhage in either group [23]. The balloon deflates slowly during succeeding months but is effectively retained through a fibrotic reaction in the wall of the vena cava.

Clinical experience with 60 patients has shown no mortality associated with use of the balloon [23]. Complications reported with an earlier design included embolization of a balloon remnant and an unstable balloon that necessitated surgical removal. Recurrent thromboembolism has not been reported. Persistent lower extremity edema ocurred in nine of 25 patients not anticoagulated at the time of occlusion and in four of 29 who were anticoagulated. Long term follow-up of 45 patients showed no edema in 36, five with no edema but wearing elastic stockings, three with mild to moderate edema without elastic stockings, and one with severe edema.

Critique of Transvenous Devices

The three devices described above represent those currently in clinical use for the prevention of pulmonary thromboembolism. They are effective in the control of recurrent thromboembolism and their associated morbidity is acceptable as compared with the risks of alternative forms of treatment (Table 1). The designs of these devices permit accommodation to a range of caval diameters, and therefore an exact filter size is unnecessary.

The devices, however, all require a surgical procedure to expose the internal jugular or femoral vein since the large caliber of the devices necessitates a venotomy. The patient is usually conscious but immo-

Table 1. Results of clinical studies of the transvenous devices currently used

Device type	No. in series	Device migration (%)	Recurrent embolism (%)	Patency rate (%)
Mobin-Uddin	2562	0.4	0.5	40
Kimray-Greenfield	76	0	2.6	97
Hunter balloon	60	3	0	0

bilized during the dissection, resulting in considerable discomfort. There is a risk of air embolism during insertion of the device through the venotomy. The devices must be guided through the right side of the heart and directed away from the hepatic and renal veins, but the delivery systems are difficult to steer. Extrusion or disengagement of the device is relatively easy once it is in the inferior vena cava.

It is also not possible to ensure that the filters will release into the vena cava lumen properly oriented in relation to the long axis of the vena cava (Figs. 4 and 5). Commonly they tilt to the side or posteriorly, the latter being difficult to detect on the standard frontal projection. Such malpositioned filters are less efficient in their ability to capture emboli [35]. Proximal migration of devices, which has been reported with the Mobin-Uddin and Hunter devices, remains a concern. Distal migration, which is of relatively little clinical significance, has also been encountered with both filters. Thrombus, demonstrated on the upper surface of these devices by venography and at autopsy, remains a potential source of recurrent emboli [35]. Complete occlusion of the inferior vena cava, as occurs with the Hunter balloon and sometimes with filters (Fig. 6), seems inherently undesirable since the large collateral channels that are likely to develop may allow passage of lethal emboli [12].

An Experimental Percutaneous Transcatheter Approach

The possibility of delivering a filtering device into the inferior vena cava without surgery, employing a regular angiographic catheter has tantalized many. Such a device could be introduced through a catheter inserted percutaneously by the standard Seldinger technique. The same catheter is commonly used to establish the angiographic diagnosis of pulmonary embolism or venous thrombosis. Thus the diagnostic and therapeutic procedures are combined, providing immediate protection against recurrent pulmonary emboli.

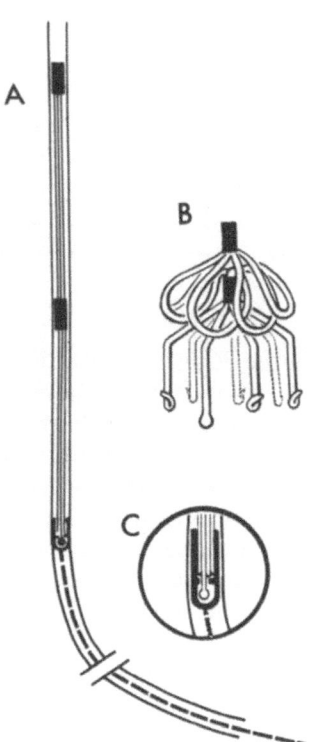

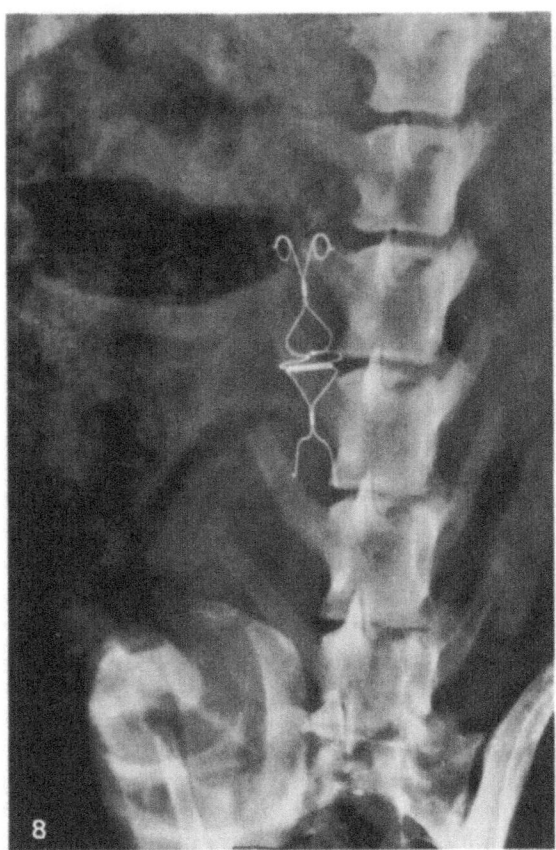

Fig. 7A–C. Nitinol inferior vena cava filter. A Straight wires loaded into a standard angiographic catheter at room temperature. B Filter configuration at body temperature after delivery into the inferior vena cava. C Detail of junction between filter and delivery guide wire.

Fig. 8. Experimental Nitinol filter. An earlier design delivered into the inferior vena cava of a dog.

The authors have developed and are currently investigating such a device made of a remarkable thermal shape-memory alloy [36] (Fig. 7). The special property of this alloy, Nitinol, enables the device to exist as a set of thin straight wires at room temperature which becomes transformed into a complex predetermined filter shape at body temperature. The filter shape is imprinted into the "memory" of the wires by winding them onto a jig and annealing them in a furnace. On cooling, the wires are removed and straightened. In its straightened form the filter may be readily passed through a standard angiographic catheter perfused with cool saline. As it is extruded into the inferior vena cava and warmed to body temperature, the device reverts to the filter shape and locks into place. Several designs have been successfully tested in dogs and have been shown to be effective in arresting even small emboli (Fig. 8). The major advantage of this device over others currently in use is that it does not require any surgical dissection or venotomy. It can be passed through the same small-bore catheter used for pulmonary angiography or venacavography, and it is anticipated that the diagnostic procedure and placement of the device, if indicated,

will be combined. Research is currently in progress to study the physical characteristics and bioacceptability of these filters and to develop an inferior vena cava filter and delivery system suitable for clinical use.

Transvenous Embolectomy

Many patients with massive thromboembolism die within the first hour. Those that survive this acute period rarely die of that particular embolic episode. When massive thromboembolism has been demonstrated by pulmonary angiography, the clinician must decide whether to ignore that embolus and treat the patient prophylactically by anticoagulants or venous interruption, whether to use thrombolytic drugs such as urokinase or streptokinase to promote clot lysis, or whether to recommend operative removal of the embolus. Sabiston's indication for pulmonary embolectomy is persistent and refractory hypotension despite adequate vasopressor and oxygen therapy. One to two hours of conservative therapy is advocated, depending on the severity of the patient's clinical con-

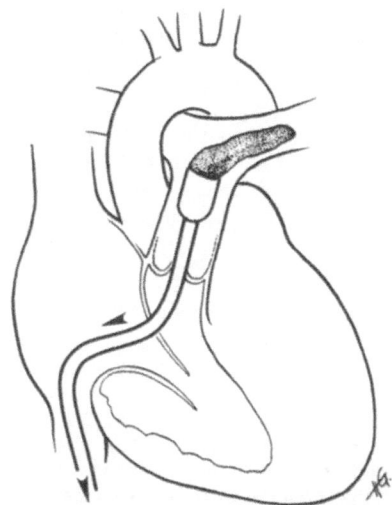

Fig. 9. Greenfield transvenous embolectomy device, consisting of a steerable catheter and suction cup. The thrombus is being withdrawn from a pulmonary artery while suction is maintained.

dition. If supportive measures can maintain a systolic pressure of 60–80 mm Hg, then pulmonary embolectomy can be deferred, particularly if the patient's renal and cerebral function is maintained [37]. Open pulmonary embolectomy using cardiopulmonary bypass [38] has high mortality (50–60%) and high morbidity, including pulmonary hemorrhage.

In an attempt to improve the prognosis of massive thromboembolism, Greenfield [39] has described a transvenous technique for pulmonary embolectomy (Fig. 9). His device consists of a 100-cm steerable catheter with a radiopaque plastic suction cup attached to the tip. Suction can be applied through the catheter, or contrast can be injected. Following identification of a pulmonary embolus a femoral venotomy is performed, and the device is inserted and guided to the occluded pulmonary artery. Part of the embolus is aspirated into the cup, and the catheter is then withdrawn while holding the embolus by continuous suction until it is delivered through the venotomy. Multiple retrievals may be necessary if the embolus cannot be withdrawn intact. This is continued until there is a significant drop in the mean pulmonary arterial pressure to normal values (20 mm Hg), as measured with a Swan-Ganz catheter [10]. Following removal of the emboli, an inferior vena cava filter is inserted to prevent further episodes.

Greenfield performed transvenous embolectomy on 12 patients who had suffered a pulmonary embolism and remained in shock despite vasopressive therapy. All were shown to have had occlusion of more than 50% of the pulmonary vascular bed. In one patient no clot could be retrieved, and in two others only small fragments could be removed; it was felt

that the failure to remove the embolus was caused by its adherence to the wall of the artery. Two deaths were reported, the first occurring before the catheter could be manipulated into the pulmonary artery. The second death followed successful removal of emboli, when the patient developed an exsanguinating hemoptysis after inflation of the Swan-Ganz catheter. Other complications included wound hematomas, pulmonary infarction, thrombophlebitis, and hemorrhagic pleural effusion.

While Greenfield's initial reports are promising, it should be emphasized that the role of transvenous embolectomy in the treatment of massive thromboembolism has not yet been defined. There is a general belief that an initial trial of non-operative management is warranted in the vast majority of patients with massive embolism. Most patients will recover because of spontaneous or stimulated thrombolysis or fragmentation and distal migration of the embolus.

Conclusion

Transvenous control of pulmonary embolism, initiated barely 10 years ago, has undergone rapid development and gained widespread acceptance. The effectiveness of transvenous devices has led to a broadening of the indications for their use. It should be stressed that placement of these devices is still associated with an appreciable complication rate and that the prevention of further peripheral thrombosis by anticoagulant therapy is usually sufficient. However, in cases in which anticoagulants are contraindicated or have been ineffective and the possibility of recurrent pulmonary thromboembolism is high, a device placed in the inferior vena cava has saved many lives and has reduced morbidity. Transvenous inferior vena cava interruption is now superseding traditional surgical approaches in many centers. We anticipate future refinements in filter design and delivery techniques to accomplish the desired goal of venous interruption more simply and effectively and with even lower morbidity, mortality, and cost. We also envision advances in the transvenous removal of emboli from the lungs.

References

1. Freiman, D.G., Suyemotto, J., Wessler, S.: Frequency of pulmonary thromboembolism in man. N. Engl. J. Med. 272:1278–1280, 1965
2. Simon, M., Sacks, B.A.: Pulmonary embolism. In: Surgical Radiology, edited by J.E. Teplick and M.E. Haskin. Philadelphia, W.B. Saunders, 1980
3. Dalen, J.E., Alpert, J.S.: Natural history of pulmonary embolism. Prog. Cardiovasc. Dis. 17:259–270, 1975

4. Gardner, A.M., Askew, A.R., Harse, H.R. Wilmshurst, C.C., Turner, M.J.: Partial occlusion of the inferior vena cava in the prevention of fatal pulmonary embolism. Surg. Gynecol. Obstet. 138:17–22, 1974

5. Sasahara, A.A., Cannilla, J.E., Morse, R.L., Sidd, J.J., Tremblay, G.M.: Clinical and physiologic studies in pulmonary thromboembolism. Am. J. Cardiol. 20:10–20, 1967

6. Thomas, M.L., Andress, M.R., Browse, N.L., Fletcher, E.W.L., Phillips, J.D., Pin, H.P., McAllister, N., Stephenson, R.H., Tange, K.: Phlebography in the prevention of recurrent pulmonary embolism: Technique and value. Am. J. Roentgenol. 110:725–733, 1970

7. Fits, W.T., Lehr, H.B., Bitner, R.L., Spelman, J.: An analysis of 950 fatal injuries. Surgery 56:663–668, 1964

8. Fullen, W.D., Miller, E.H., Steele, W.F., McDonough, J.J.: Prophylactic vena cava interruption in hip fractures. J. Trauma 13:403–410, 1973

9. Rhodes, G.R., Dixon, R.H., Silver, D.: Heparin induced thrombocytopenia. Ann. Surg. 186:752–758, 1977

10. Greenfield, L.J., Zocco, J.J.: Intraluminal management of acute massive pulmonary thromboembolism. J. Thorac. Cardiovasc. Surg. 77:402–410, 1979

11. O'Neill, E.E.: Ligation of the inferior vena cava in the prevention and treatment of pulmonary embolism. N. Engl. J. Med. 232:641–646, 1945

12. Edwards, E.A., Dexter, L., Donahue, W.C.: Recurrent pulmonary embolism as a remediable cause of heart failure. Geriatrics 16:423–432, 1961

13. DeWeese, M.D., Hunter, D.C.: A vena caval filter for the prevention of pulmonary emboli. Bull. Soc. Int. Chir. 17:117–125, 1958

14. Spencer, F.C.: An experimental evaluation of partitioning of the inferior vena cava to prevent pulmonary embolism. Surg. Forum 10:680–684, 1959

15. Mozes, M., Antebi, E.: A simple method for plication of the inferior vena cava. Surg. Gynecol. Obstet. 125:362–364, 1967

16. Adams, J.T., DeWeese, J.A.: Experimental and clinical evaluation of partial vein interruption in the prevention of pulmonary emboli. Surgery 57:82–102, 1965

17. Bernstein, E.F.: The role of operative inferior vena caval interruption in the management of venous thromboembolism. World J. Surg. 22:61–71, 1978

18. Rosenthal, D., Cossman, D., Matsumoto, G., Callow, A.D.: Prophylactic interruption of the inferior vena cava. A retrospective evaluation. Am. J. Surg. 137:389–393, 1979

19. Blumenberg, R.M., Gelfand, M.L.: Long-term follow-up of vena caval clips and umbrellas. Am. J. Surg. 134:205–213, 1977

20. Eichelter, P., Schenk, W.G., Jr.: Prophylaxis of pulmonary embolism: A new experimental approach with initial results. Arch. Surg. 97:348–356, 1968

21. Moser, K.M., Harsany, P.G., Harvey-Smith, W., Durante, P.L., Giuson, M.: Reversible interruption of the inferior vena cava by means of a balloon catheter: Preliminary report. J. Thorac. Cardiovasc. Surg. 62:205–213, 1971

22. Pate, J.W., Melvin, D., Cheek, R.C.: A new form of vena caval interruption. Ann. Surg. 169:873–880, 1969

23. Hunter, J.A., Dye, W.S., Javid, H., Najafi, H., Goldin, M.D., Serry, C.: Permanent transvenous balloon occlusion of the inferior vena cava. Ann. Surg. 186:491–499, 1977

24. Mobin-Uddin, K., Utley, J.R., Bryant, L.R.: The inferior vena cava umbrella filter. Progr. Cardiovasc. Dis. 17:391–399, 1975

25. Greenfield, L.J., Zocco, J., Wilk, J., Schroeder, T.M., Elkins, R.C.: Clinical experience with the Kimray Greenfield vena caval filter. Ann. Surg. 185:692–698, 1977

26. McConnell, D., Mulder, D., Buckberg, G.: The placement of vena cava umbrella filters: The value of phlebography. Arch. Surg. 108:789–791, 1974

27. Scott, J.H., Anderson, C.L., Shanker, P.S.: Septicemia from infected caval "umbrella" (letter). JAMA 243:1133–1134, 1980

28. Mobin-Uddin, K., Martinez, L.O., Jude, J.R.: A vena cava filter for the prevention of pulmonary embolus. Surg. Forum 18:209–211, 1967

29. Mobin-Uddin, K., McLean, R., Jude, J.R.: A new catheter technique of interruption of the inferior vena cava for prevention of pulmonary embolism. Am. Surg. 35:889–894, 1969

30. Steer, M., Adelson, J., Glotzer, D.J., Skillman, J.J., Simon, M., Salzman, E.: Thromboembolism after insertion of the Mobin-Uddin Caval Filter. Surgery (in press)

31. Mobin-Uddin, K.: Invited commentary. World J. Surg. 2:55–57, 1978

32. Greenfield, L.J., McCurdy, J.R., Brown, P.P., Elkins, R.C.: A new intracaval filter permitting continued flow and resolution of emboli. Surgery 73:599–606, 1973

33. Wingerd, M., Bernhard, V.M., Maddison, F., Towne, J.B.: Comparison of caval filters in the management of venous thromboembolism. Arch. Surg. 113:1264–1271, 1978

34. Hunter, J.A., Sessions, R., Buenger, R.: Experimental balloon obstruction of the inferior vena cava. Ann. Surg. 171:315–320, 1970

35. Fullen, W.D., McDonough, J.J., Altemeier, W.A.: Clinical experience with vena caval filters. Arch. Surg. 106:582–587, 1973

36. Simon, M., Kaplow, R., Salzman, E., Freiman, D.: A vena cava filter using thermal shape memory alloy: Experimental aspects. Radiology 125:89–94, 1977

37. Sabiston, D.G., Wolfe, W.G.: Pulmonary embolectomy. In: Pulmonary Thromboembolism, edited by K.M. Moser and M. Stein. Chicago, Year Book Medical Publishers. 1973, pp. 327–338

38. Scannell, J.G.: The surgical management of acute massive pulmonary embolism. Progr. Cardiovasc. Dis. 9:488–474, 1967

39. Greenfield, L.J., Peyton, M.D., Brown, P.P., Elkins, R.C.: Transvenous management of pulmonary embolic disease. Ann. Surg. 180:461–468, 1974

Comment

Transvenous Management of Pulmonary Embolism and Technical Aspects of Filters

Ernest J. Ferris

Department of Radiology, University of Arkansas for Medical Sciences, Little Rock, Arkansas, USA

Drs. Simon and Palestrant have concisely, but thoroughly, reviewed the use of transvenous devices in the prevention of pulmonary embolism.

In general, I would agree with their analysis of indications for the procedure. When evaluating pulmonary embolism, I attempt, when feasible, to evaluate the venous source. Furthermore, a semi-quantitative estimate is made of both venous thrombosis (if found) and the pulmonary embolism.

If a patient suffers even several bouts of hemodynamically mild pulmonary embolism from, for example, small thrombi in the calf, I may hesitate to recommend transvenous interruption, particularly in a young person, even if heparin and streptase therapy have not been effective. There are times, however, when a "few small emboli" do provoke severe physiologic and hemodynamic changes, and hence may require aggressive therapy, such as the placement of a transvenous device. Conversely, in some patients with cardiopulmonary insufficiency, one often recommends transvenous interruption after a single large embolus or a hemodynamically significant embolus of even relatively small size. In such a case, the condition of the host, rather than the disease entity per se, is the determinant.

In their section on insertion of the transvenous device, the authors stress the importance of renal vein identification for the strategic positioning of the device immediately below the lowermost renal vein. This important principle carries the implication that the vascular radiologist should be involved in the procedure. All too often I have seen devices placed crudely by the inexperienced who have used as a landmark a vertebral body, that was inappropriately selected by renal vein position estimates derived from excretory urography.

Although the device is almost invariably positioned below the renal veins, there are some exceptions. I had the opportunity to insert a Mobin-Uddin filter into the inferior vena cava in a patient with non-ascent of kidneys, i.e., a pelvic "clump" kidney. No change in renal function occurred in the immediate post-procedural period, and six-month follow-up demonstrated normal renal function. Fortunately the inferior vena cava below the filter remained patent. It is likely, although unproven, that collateral venous pelvic routes would develop in the event of gradual caval occlusion secondary to filter "stasis."

As Drs. Simon and Palestrant have discussed, the Mobin-Uddin filter has a low patency rate (approximately 40%). In the initial procedures I performed with this filter, I noted frequent early occlusion with propogating thrombi below and, to a lesser degree, above the device. Therefore, in the last 103 procedures I performed, I attempted to improve flow in the immediate post-procedure period by elevating the legs and (when not contraindicated) employing elastic stockings. If possible, heparin administration was instituted some 10–12 hours after insertion of the device and maintained for a minimum of ten days. Although I have not been able to follow most of the patients because of logistical reasons, it is my impression that the clinical incidence of caval occlusion has been much lower in these last cases, probably reflecting a higher patency rate.

In my series of 113 patients in whom a transvenous Mobin-Uddin filter was inserted, three patients died after almost immediate massive thrombosis above and below the filter and recurrent pulmonary embolism. The three patients had malignancies of various types with disseminated intravascular coagulation.

Address reprint requests to: E.J. Ferris, M.D., University of Arkansas for Medical Sciences, Little Rock, AR 72205 USA

The Nitinol (Simon) wire, which, as discussed in this paper, reshapes itself at body temperature, is an ingenious development that holds great promise for clinical application.

Finally, since we are inserting foreign bodies into the vascular system, and there has been at least one reported case of filter infection [1], some thought should be given to the use of prophylactic antibiotics. We should probably approach this problem as our cardiac surgical colleagues approach the insertion of artifical heart valves. If we insert the devices, we should follow the patients and be involved in initiation and maintenance of medical aids referrable to the procedure. In other words, our involvement cannot be merely technical or consultatory, but occasionally it must dictate direct and continuous patient care and follow-up!

Reference

1. Scott, J.H., Anderson, C.L., Shankar, P.S.: Septicemia from infected caval "umbrella" (letters). JAMA 243:1133–1134, 1980

Practical Points on Transvenous Insertion of Inferior Vena Cava Filters

Robert A. Novelline

Department of Radiology, Harvard Medical School and Massachusetts General Hospital, Boston, Massachusetts, USA

Abstract. During the transvenous insertion of Kimray-Greenfield (KG) and Mobin-Uddin (MU) inferior vena cava filters at the Massachusetts General Hospital, several problems have been encountered and successfully resolved. The author offers suggestions for dealing with small or spastic internal jugular veins, prominent eustachian valves (valves of the inferior vena cava), congenital variations in the inferior vena cava, inferior vena cava thrombi, and filters that have been placed too low or too high. In addition, methods are described for directing the KG filter with gravity, identifying the lowest renal vein with a selective catheter, inserting the KG filter from a femoral venous route, assuring proper seating of an MU filter, and confirming filter position following placement.

Key words: Embolism, pulmonary — Vena cava, transvenous interruption — Interventional radiology.

At the Massachusetts General Hospital we have inserted 61 inferior vena cava filters: 27 Mobin-Uddin (MU) and 34 Kimray-Greenfield (KG) filters. (We have not used the Hunter balloon.) In our series there was no mortality and only minimal morbidity, and the devices have proved lifesaving in patients with thromboembolic disease who could not be anticoagulated and who were at high risk for general anesthesia and surgical inferior vena cava clipping.

The KG filter is preferred to the MU device because with the KG filter there is a higher rate of inferior vena cava patency and a lower incidence of venous stasis syndromes and recurrent pulmonary embolism [1–3]. The KG filter has an added advan-

tage in that it can also be inserted from a femoral vein with a special catheter-carrier (applicator).

While we are currently using the KG filter almost exclusively, the MU applicator has certain advantages over the KG applicator, and MU filters are still inserted at our hospital when we are unable to advance a KG applicator into the inferior vena cava for filter extrusion. The MU applicator has a smaller capsule (7-mm diameter, 32-mm length) than the KG jugular vein applicator capsule (8-mm diameter, 55-mm length), and the "bullet nose" tip of the loaded MU applicator slides more easily through tortuous veins and bypasses venous valves better than the "cut-off open cylinder" tip of the KG applicator. The MU applicator can also be directed more easily since its stylet can be easily bent to produce a slight curve on the distal applicator for torque control.

Technical Considerations

In the insertion of inferior vena cava filters a number of technical considerations – including possible anatomic variations as well as the characteristics of the filters themselves – must be taken into account.

The Small, Spastic, or Tortuous Jugular Vein

It may not be possible to advance a KG applicator capsule through a small, spastic, or tortuous jugular vein. We, unlike Greenfield [4], have not been successful in using a Fogarty catheter to dilate such veins so that they would then accept a KG applicator. However, we have been able to pass the bullet-nose, smaller-sized MU applicator capsule through jugular venous routes that could not be negotiated with the KG system. In patients in whom an MU applicator could not be advanced through the right jugular ve-

Address reprint request to: R.A. Novelline, M.D., Department of Radiology, Massachusetts General Hospital, Fruit Street, Boston, MA 02114, USA

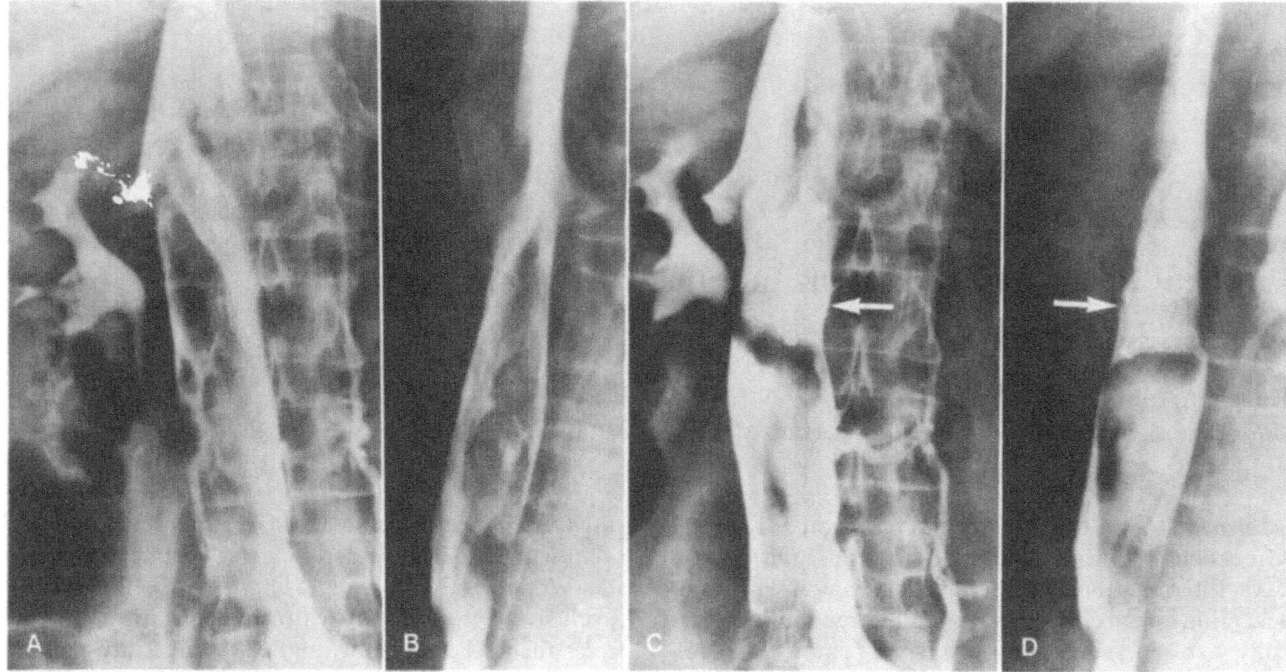

Fig. 1 A–D. A and **B** Anteroposterior and lateral views of the initial inferior vena cavagram of a patient with caval thrombus extending from the right iliac veins. **C** and **D** An MU filter is shown in place in the infrarenal cava in the same patient (*arrows*). The filter had been extruded and opened just above the level of the thrombus. and the thrombus pushed down and filter appropriately positioned in the open position prior to separation from the applicator stylet. This patient did well without recurrent pulmonary embolism.

nous route, the jugular venotomy was closed and a KG filter inserted via a femoral venotomy.

In one patient, use of a left jugular approach was successful for inferior vena cava filter insertion; however, it was only with great difficulty that the tortuous left innominate vein was negotiated. The patient noted chest discomfort for three days following the procedure and mediastinal widening, consistent with venous bleeding into the mediastinum, was present for several weeks afterwards. We do not recommend the left jugular route for filter insertion.

The Prominent Eustachian Valve

The KG jugular vein applicator is difficult to direct, and in several patients it was not possible to advance it into the inferior vena cava from the right atrium around a prominent eustachian valve (valve of the inferior vena cava). In each case we were able to advance an MU applicator into the inferior vena cava by curving the distal applicator stylet slightly; with the better torque control of the MU applicator, we were able to circumvent the prominent eustachian valve. The other option would have been to insert a KG filter through a femoral route, but this would have required a second venotomy.

Inferior Vena Cava Thrombus

Thrombus in the inferior vena cava does not necessarily obviate filter placement in the cava. Figure 1 shows a patient with a large thrombus extending from the right iliac vein to the level of the renal veins. The top of the thrombus was pushed down with a previously extruded MU filter. After the opened umbrella filter was advanced caudally to an appropriate infrarenal site, pushing the thrombus below it, it was released from the applicator stylet. This technique has also been used with a partially inflated Hunter balloon inserted from the jugular route [10].

Directing the KG Applicator with Gravity

Although the KG jugular vein applicator is floppy and lacks torque control, the heavy metal capsule at its distal end favors dependent positions within the patient. This feature may be used to improve directability. In a recent case, a jugular KG applicator would only advance down the right renal vein of a patient with a ptotic right kidney; in the supine position it was impossible to advance the KG applicator down the infrarenal cava. The applicator capsule was withdrawn to the suprarenal cava and the patient

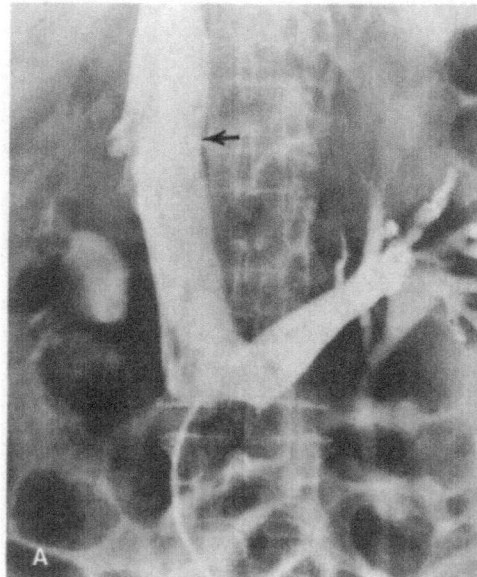
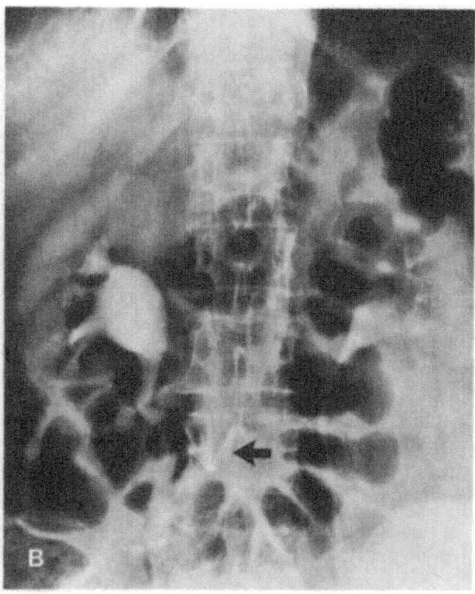

Fig. 2A and B. A Left renal venogram in a patient with a retroaortic left renal vein. The retroaortic left renal vein enters the cava at the level of L3; renal veins normally join the cava at the level of the L1–L2 interspace (*arrow*). **B** Mobin-Uddin filter correctly positioned below the level of the retroaortic left renal vein (*arrow*).

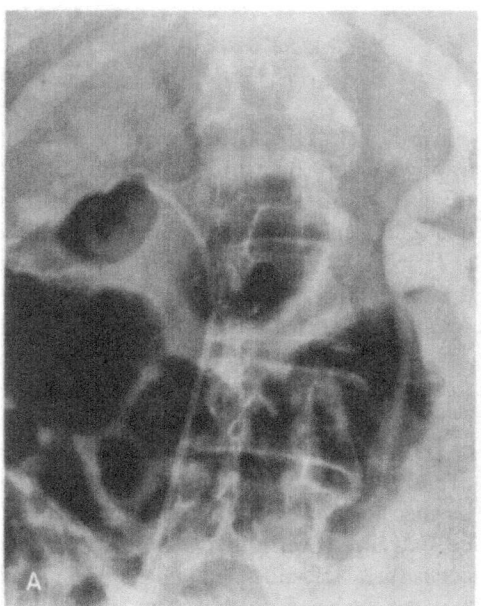
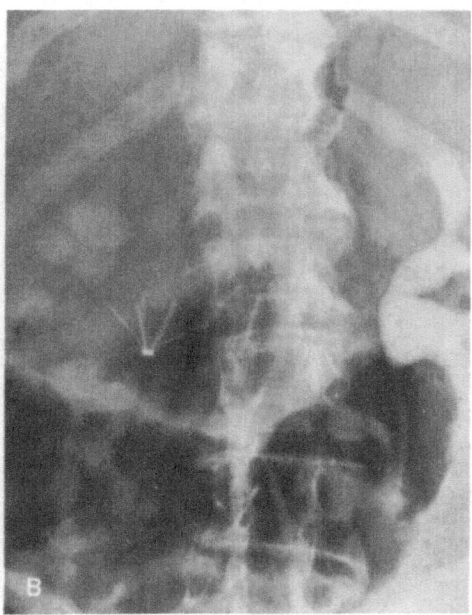

Fig. 3A and B. A Selective catheter positioned in the right renal vein to identify the level of the lowest renal vein before filter extrusion. **B** Mobin-Uddin filter appropriately positioned in the same patient.

was turned on his left side. Because the metal capsule favors dependent positions, it swung down from the orifice of the right renal vein to the infrarenal cava where it was advanced to an excellent position for filter extrusion. We have used this technique in four patients.

Inserting a KG Filter from the Femoral Route

The femoral venous route for KG filter insertion has been used in patients with tracheostomies, recent neck surgery, neck muscle contractures, and small jugular veins. The right femoral approach is preferable be-

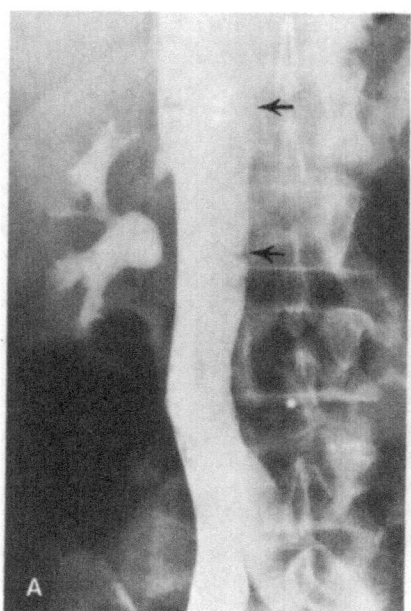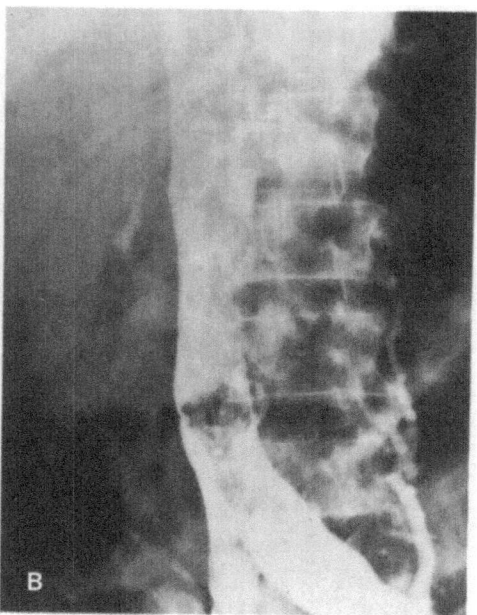

Fig. 4A and B. A Mobin-Uddin filter inadvertently placed too low (at the level of the L3–L4 interspace) in a patient with two left renal veins (*arrows*). **B** Inferior vena cavogram of the same patient seven days later, after a clinical episode of recurrent pulmonary embolism. Thrombus, which had become the source of the recurrent pulmonary embolism, can be seen on top of the filter. This patient was treated by surgical ligation of the inferior vena cava above the level of the thrombosed filter; placement of a second filter above the thrombosed filter would have been an alternative approach.

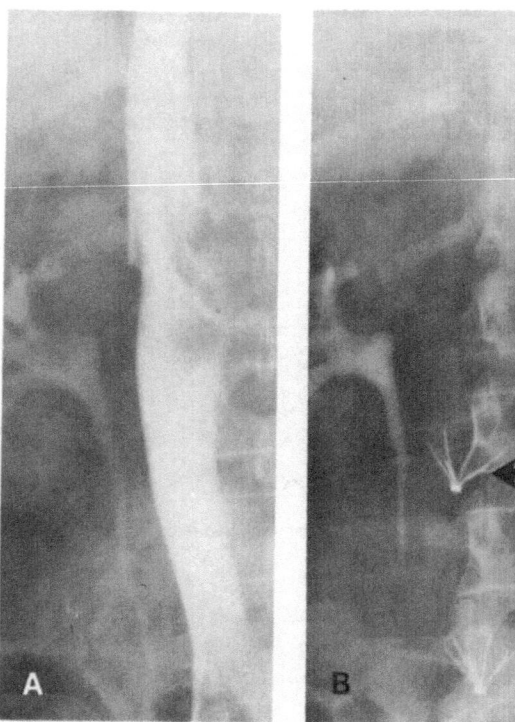

Fig. 5A and B. A Normal inferior vena cava in a patient scheduled for filter placement. **B** The first filter had been inadvertently placed too low at the level of L4. A second filter was placed above it just below the level of the renal veins (*arrows*).

cause it is easier to negotiate the KG femoral vein applicator up the more direct right iliac venous route than through the more tortuous left iliac veins. A useful feature of the femoral KG applicator is that a J or other guidewire can be advanced ahead of the applicator system (through the carrier and filter) to guide it through tortuous iliac veins. After the wire has been advanced into the inferior vena cava, the applicator system can be slid over the wire to an appropriate position in the cava for filter extrusion.

If a patient has a left-sided inferior vena cava draining into the left renal vein, a KG filter should be inserted via the left femoral vein route. It would be extremely difficult if not impossible to place a filter in a left-sided cava from a jugular route. If the patient has a double cava, with the left-sided cava draining into the left renal vein, two filters should be placed, the left-sided filter via a left femoral venotomy and the right-sided filter by either a right femoral or right jugular vein route.

Congenital Variations of the Inferior Vena Cava

Cava filters should be inserted in an angiography suite with good fluoroscopic control and filming capability for cavography before and after filter placement.

Cavography is always performed before filter placement to identify any congenital variations in the inferior vena cava or renal veins that would affect the site of filter extrusion [5–7]. Ideally cavography is performed via a left femoral vein catheterization so that duplicated or left-sided inferior vena cava will not be overlooked. The cavogram may also reveal accessory renal veins joining the cava at a level lower than the L1–L2 interspace where the main renal veins are usually located. One common variation is a retroaortic left renal vein that enters the cava two to three vertebral interspaces below the main left renal vein (Fig. 2). To be certain that accessory renal veins are not missed at cavography, they are searched for with a curved selective catheter.

Identifying the Lowest Renal Vein for Accurate Filter Placement Position

Especially with MU filters, accurate placement just below the renal veins is imperative. To pinpoint the exact location of the lowest renal vein at the time of filter extrusion, the tip of a curved selective catheter is positioned in the lowest renal vein via a transfemoral venous catheterization (Fig. 3). The applicator capsule is appropriately positioned fluoroscopically, using the selective catheter as a landmark. The selective catheter is withdrawn into an iliac vein just before filter extrusion.

Filter Placed too Low

An MU filter placed too low in the infrarenal cava is likely to become a source of recurrent pulmonary emboli (Fig. 4). If a low position inadvertently occurs, a second filter may be placed above in the immediate infrarenal position through the same venotomy (Fig. 5). Exact positioning of a KG filter is not so critical and if positioned low in the infrarenal cava, it is not necessary to place another above. However, if a KG filter is inadvertently placed in an iliac vein, then a second filter should be placed above.

Filter Placed too High (Above the Renal Veins)

There is considerable controversy over methods for dealing with an IVC filter that is placed above the renal veins. While some physicians believe that such filters should all be removed surgically, KG filters have a high patency rate, and uncomplicated suprarenal placement has been reported [4]. A KG filter prematurely released high in the inferior vena cava

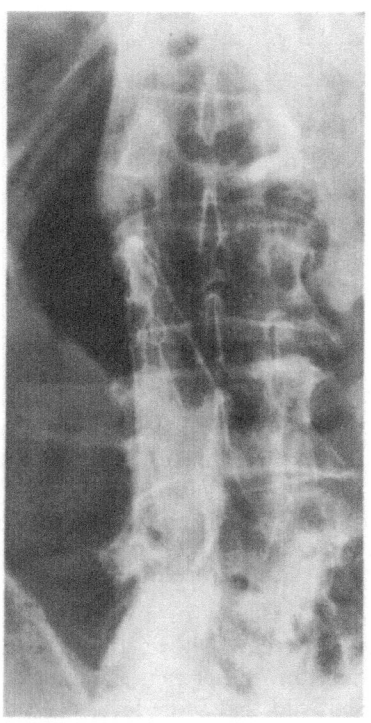

Fig. 6. A KG filter tilted 15° from the vertical axis of the patient, yet properly positioned within the inferior vena cava. Positioning of inferior vena cava filters should be assessed by inferior vena cavography rather than by plain films. In this patient the inferior vena cava is also tilted 15° at the level of the filter.

should not be pushed caudally with the applicator capsule. As the tines of the filter point caudad, pushing an extruded KG filter may result in caval perforation, as has been reported by Phillips et al. [8].

The tines of an MU filter point cephalad and this filter has been successfully pushed down after extrusion from the applicator capsule. In a report by Mobin-Uddin et al. [9] this maneuver was performed in three patients by pushing downward on the filter with the applicator capsule. In two of these, a second filter was implanted proximal to the first, which had become tilted.

Assuring Proper Seating of a MU Filter

After an MU filter has been extruded from the applicator capsule, and before unscrewing the applicator stylet from the filter, fluoroscopic observations should be made while tugging slightly on the applicator stylet to be sure that all six tines are engaged in the cava wall. If not, the tines should be opened further by pressing on the filter with the applicator capsule while continuing to tug on the applicator stylet. This technique will spread the tines over a wider area. In some patients it may be necessary to adjust the filter position by slightly advancing the applicator stylet and capsule together. The applicator stylet should not be unscrewed from the filter until the filter is properly seated. A KG filter is not screwed onto the pusher stylet, and once the applicator capsule has been lifted off the filter and the filter extruded, no further adjustments are required or possible.

Confirming Filter Position Following Placement

Cavography should always be performed following extrusion of MU or KG filters to insure proper filter position. The relationship of the filter to the inferior vena cava can be best assessed, and malposition or caval perforation by filter tines identified, on cavography. Plain films alone may be misleading. Figure 6 illustrates a KG filter tilted 15° from the vertical axis of the patient. Injection of a contrast medium into the inferior vena cava shows that the filter is not malpositioned, but rather that the inferior vena cava is also tilted 15° at that same level.

Medication

Because the tines of both MU and KG filters are engaged in the wall of the inferior vena cava, patients should not be treated with streptokinase or other thrombolytic agents after filter placement since this may cause severe retroperitoneal bleeding. Ideally patients with caval filters should be treated with anti-

coagulants for several weeks, beginning 24 hours after filter placement. This is usually not feasible, however, because patients selected for filter placement are usually those in whom anticoagulants are contraindicated.

References

1. Wingerd, M., Bernhard, V.M., Maddison, F., Towne, J.B.: Comparison of caval filters in the management of venous thromboembolism. Arch. Surg. 113:1264–1271, 1978
2. Cimochowski, G.E., Evans, R.H., Zarins, C.K., Lu, C.T., DeMeester, T.R.: Greenfield filter versus Mobin-Uddin umbrella: The continuing quest for the ideal method of vena caval interruption. J. Thorac. Cardiovasc. Surg. 79:358–365, 1980
3. Berland, L.L., Maddison, F.E., Bernhard V.M.: Radiologic follow-up of vena cava filter devices. Am. J. Roentgenol. 34:1047–1052, 1980
4. Greenfield, L.J.: The surgeon at work: Technical considerations for insertion of vena caval filters. Surg. Gynecol. Obstet. 148:422–426, 1979
5. Gray, R.K., Buckberg, G.D., Grollman, J.H., Jr: The importance of inferior vena cavography in placement of the Mobin-Uddin vena caval filter. Radiology 106:277–280, 1973
6. Riggs, O.E.: Vena cavography relative to umbrella filter placement. Radiology 105:450–451, 1972
7. Fee, H.J., McAvoy, J.H., O'Connell, T.X.: Treatment and prevention of Mobin-Uddin umbrella misplacement. Arch. Surg. 113:331–332, 1978
8. Phillips, M.R., Widrich, W.C., Johnson, W.C.: Perforation of the inferior vena cava by the Kimray Greenfield filter. Surgery 87:233–235, 1980
9. Mobin-Uddin, K., Utley, J.R., Bryant, L.R.: The inferior vena cava umbrella filter. Progr. Cardiovasc. Dis. 17:391–399, 1975
10. Hunter J.A., Sessions, R., Petasnick, J.: Therapeutic balloon occlusion of the inferior vena cava. JAMA 234:1034–1036, 1975

Comment

Filter Interruption of the Inferior Vena Cava

Ernest J. Ferris

Department of Radiology, University of Arkansas for Medical Sciences, Little Rock, Arkansas, USA

The introduction of inferior vena cava filters via the transvenous route seems relatively easy in uncomplicated cases. However, as pointed out by Dr. Novelline, there are many inherent difficulties arising from variations in anatomy, pathologic alterations within the cava, abnormalities secondary to malposition of

Address reprint requests to: E.J. Ferris, M.D., Department of Radiology, University of Arkansas for Medical Sciences, Little Rock, AR 72205, USA

filters, etc., that require different technical approaches. It therefore behooves the vascular radiologist to be able to cope, not only with standard approaches, but also with the exceptions to the rule. In this regard Dr. Novelline has outlined in a superb fashion alternative approaches in a host of different situations. The logical and most important conclusion of this paper is that it is the vascular radiologist who should directly assume responsibility for the tranvenous insertion of inferior vena cava filters.